CONCORD FREE PUBLIC LIBRARY

P9-DDN-628

4 14 DAYS NOT RENEWABLE

the**facts**

Stroke

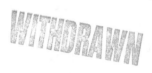

WITHDRAWN

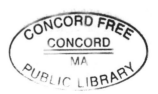

CONCORD FREE
CONCORD
MA
PUBLIC LIBRARY

AUG 15 '08

→ also available in the**facts** series

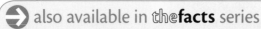

the**facts**

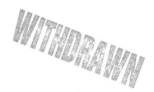

Stroke

RICHARD I. LINDLEY

Professor of Geriatric Medicine
Moran Foundation for Older Australians
University of Sydney
Australia

OXFORD
UNIVERSITY PRESS

OXFORD
UNIVERSITY PRESS

616 81
Lindley

Great Clarendon Street, Oxford OX2 6DP

Oxford University Press is a department of the University of Oxford.
It furthers the University's objective of excellence in research, scholarship,
and education by publishing worldwide in

Oxford New York

Auckland Cape Town Dar es Salaam Hong Kong Karachi
Kuala Lumpur Madrid Melbourne Mexico City Nairobi
New Delhi Shanghai Taipei Toronto

With offices in

Argentina Austria Brazil Chile Czech Republic France Greece
Guatemala Hungary Italy Japan Poland Portugal Singapore
South Korea Switzerland Thailand Turkey Ukraine Vietnam

Oxford is a registered trade mark of Oxford University Press
in the UK and in certain other countries

Published in the United States
by Oxford University Press Inc., New York

© Oxford University Press, 2008

The moral rights of the author have been asserted
Database right Oxford University Press (maker)

First edition published 2008

All rights reserved. No part of this publication may be reproduced,
stored in a retrieval system, or transmitted, in any form or by any means,
without the prior permission in writing of Oxford University Press,
or as expressly permitted by law, or under terms agreed with the appropriate
reprographics rights organization. Enquiries concerning reproduction
outside the scope of the above should be sent to the Rights Department,
Oxford University Press, at the address above

You must not circulate this book in any other binding or cover
and you must impose this same condition on any acquirer

British Library Cataloguing in Publication Data

Data available

Library of Congress Cataloguing in Publication Data

Data available

ISBN 978-0-19-921272-9 (Pbk.)

10 9 8 7 6 5 4 3 2 1

Typeset in Plantin
by Cepha Imaging Pvt. Ltd., Bangalore, India
Printed in Great Britain
on acid-free paper by
Ashford Colour Press, Gosport, Hampshire

While every effort has been made to ensure that the contents of this book are as complete, accurate
and up-to-date as possible at the date of writing, Oxford University Press is not able to give
any guarantee or assurance that such is the case. Readers are urged to take appropriately
qualified medical advice in all cases. The information in this book is intended to be useful to
the general reader, but should not be used as a means of self-diagnosis or for the prescription of
medication. The authors and the publishers do not accept responsibility or legal liability for any
errors in the text or for the misuse or misapplication of material in this book.

This book is dedicated to PAC

Contents

Acknowledgements

I would like to thank my colleagues at the University of Sydney and Sydney West Area Health Service who granted me a 2-month sabbatical in order to write this book, and my fellow geriatricians at Westmead Hospital who covered my clinical work during my absence. Many people contributed to the success of my sabbatical, including Surat Boonyakarncul and his colleagues at the Thai Stroke Society, Derick Wade, Alastair Buchan, Peter Rothwell, Veronica Murray, Bent Indredavik, Peter Sandercock, Joanna Wardlaw, Charles Warlow, Martin Dennis, Jane Collier, Ian Jordan, Mark Cousins, Rohan Grimley, Genevieve Freys, Paul Chmielnik, and my parents. My current post at the University of Sydney is supported by the Moran Foundation for Older Australians and an infrastructure grant from NSW Health.

Richard I. Lindley

Sydney 2007

1

What is stroke?

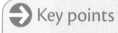

Key points

◆ Stroke is the third most common cause of death (after heart disease and cancer) in developed countries.

◆ It is a disease of the brain (*not* the heart) and is caused by a blockage or rupture of the essential blood supply.

◆ A transient ischaemic attack (TIA), or 'mini-stroke' is a major warning sign of impending major stroke and needs to be taken seriously.

◆ 'Brain attack' has been suggested as a useful new name for the first 24 hours of a stroke or TIA.

Stroke has been recognized for thousands of years and is the third most common cause of death in developed countries (after heart attacks and all cancers combined). Although it can affect people of all ages, it is most common in old age. Perhaps because of the association between stroke and old age, or terminal disease, it has not had the profile of other perhaps less serious or rarer disorders and thus is less well known to the general public. However, stroke is so common that most people will know someone who has had a stroke or have a close family member who has had a stroke.

Stroke has had a major effect on world politics as many political leaders have had a stroke or died of a stroke. Ariel Sharon, when Prime Minister of Israel, had a minor stroke in December 2005, followed by a devastating stroke a few weeks later which left him severely disabled and unfit for office. Winston Churchill had a series of strokes during his lifetime, including one (kept secret from the public in 1949) before his third and final term of office as British Prime Minister. The former American President Richard Nixon died

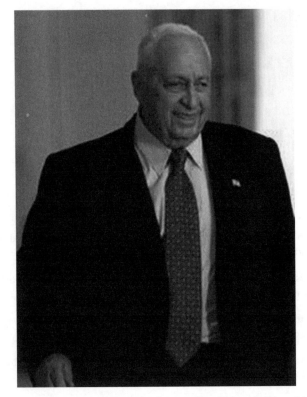

Figure 1.1 Prime Minister Ariel Sharon had two strokes which ended his political life and affected the political history of the Middle East.

of a stroke. President Dwight Eisenhower suffered a mild stroke in the Oval Office in the White House in November 1957. It is also reported that Margaret Thatcher has had a series of small strokes.

Many other famous people have also had strokes. The American actor Kirk Douglas made a remarkable recovery from a severe stroke and wrote a book about his experiences. The Australian tennis star John Newcombe also wrote about his stroke. Samuel Johnson, one of England's best known literary figures, had a stroke on the 17 June 1783. His thoughts at the time were:

> I was alarmed, and prayed God, that however he might afflict my body, he would spare my understanding. This prayer, that I might

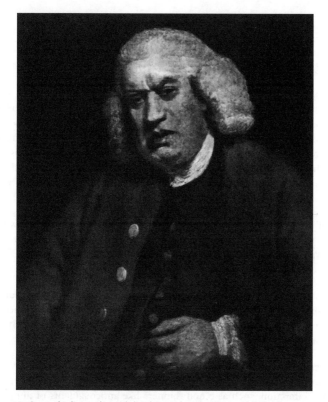

Figure 1.2 Samuel Johnson hoped that his stroke would spare his intellect.

try the integrity of my faculties, I made in Latin verse. The lines
were not very good, but I knew them not to be very good.

A stroke occurs when the blood supply to the brain is disrupted, and part of
the brain stops working. This produces sudden characteristic symptoms ranging from a rapidly fatal illness to a barely perceived loss of sensation on one
side of the body. This variability causes many problems! It is hard for the layman to understand what a stroke is (or is not) as there are so many variants. It
is also often hard for doctors and nurses to make the correct diagnosis, as
many illnesses mimic stroke. Surveys of public knowledge of stroke have
shown that this common disorder is not well understood. Many people are not
aware that the problem lies within the brain. It is certainly not the same thing
as a heart attack, which has quite different symptoms (usually severe chest
pain). Stroke is not usually accompanied by severe pain. If pain is present, it is

usually a headache and may be a sign that the stroke has been due to a brain haemorrhage.

The underlying cause of stroke

There are actually two main causes of stroke which, confusingly, can present in exactly the same manner. About 80 per cent of all strokes are due to blockage or **occlusion** of the blood supply to the brain, usually from a blood clot. Blood clots can develop along a blood vessel or may have travelled along the blood vessel from a source further away. The latter sort of blood clot is called an **embolus**. Strokes caused by occlusion of blood vessels are due to death of brain tissue, which is known as **cerebral infarction**. This type of stroke is commonly called **ischaemic stroke**.

The other main pathological cause of stroke is **brain haemorrhage**, which is caused when a blood vessel in the brain (the **cerebral artery**) leaks or bursts. This type of stroke is called **primary intracerebral haemorrhage**. About 15 per cent of strokes are of this type.

The final 5 per cent of strokes are caused by a condition called **subarachnoid haemorrhage** which has a very different presentation, assessment, and treatment from ischaemic stroke and primary intracerebral haemorrhage. It is not discussed further in this book.

A closer inspection of these causes of stroke reveal a major difficulty in the assessment and treatment of the condition. Treatments which can help prevent cerebral infarction, such as blood thinners like anticoagulants or antiplatelet medication, can sometimes cause primary intracerebral infarction. Likewise, treatments for primary intracerebral haemorrhage, such as blood clotting factors, can sometimes cause **cerebral thrombosis** (clots in the blood vessels in the brain). Therein lies the problem: there are two very different types of stroke which require very different approaches to treatment. Indeed, until the invention of the computed tomography scanner (CT scanner) in the 1970s, it was impossible to reliably distinguish cerebral infarction from primary intracerebral haemorrhage and therefore it is not surprising that successful emergency treatments for stroke have only been developed in the last 30 years.

The changing names for stroke

The Greek physician Hippocrates (about 460–370 BC) recognized stroke and called it 'apoplexy', derived from the Greek word 'apoplexia' (being struck with violence). It is likely that Hippocrates and his followers used this name for the most catastrophic of strokes, such as large primary intracerebral haemorrhages or subarachnoid haemorrhages which commonly cause loss of consciousness and can rapidly lead to death. We still describe such a rapid and severe onset of illness as 'apoplectic'. Hippocrates also recognized other types of stroke. He used the term 'partial apoplexy' to describe someone with a 'hemiparesis' – a weakness of the face, arm, and leg on one side of the body. A well-known saying of the time reflected the expected outcome from such disorders: 'It is impossible to cure a severe attack of apoplexy, and difficult to cure a mild one'. This sentiment is still held, rather inaccurately, by many doctors today.

Since the time of Hippocrates a large variety of terms have been used to describe stroke. Perhaps the most commonly used, and the least helpful, is 'cerebrovascular accident' (CVA). The term 'stroke', which has been used by the layman for several hundred years, conveys the suddenness and randomness with which it occurs, and has now become the preferred medical term.

As 'stroke' and 'transient ischaemic attack' have become the widely accepted standard medical terms, it is useful to look at their definitions.

Definition of stroke and transient ischaemic attack

Medical definition of stroke

A stroke is a clinical syndrome characterized by rapidly developing clinical symptoms and/or signs of focal, and at times global (applied to patients in deep coma and those with subarachnoid haemorrhage), loss of cerebral function, with symptoms lasting more than 24 hours or leading to death, with no apparent cause other than that of vascular origin (Hatano 1976).

The use of this definition of stroke over the past 30 years has had many advantages. The description of 'rapid onset' of neurological symptoms nicely captures the key features of stroke for healthcare professionals. In fact, this is a defining feature of vascular disease (disease of the blood vessels). A heart attack (occlusion of a coronary artery by a ruptured atherosclerotic plaque) is characterized by sudden chest pain. Arterial thrombosis of the leg is characterized by a sudden onset of a painful, pulseless, and pale leg.

Focal neurological signs, such as weakness down one side (unilateral hemiparesis) or loss of vision (unilateral loss of visual field called hemianopia), describe the common patterns of stroke symptoms that are due to the way the blood is supplied to the brain, which follows a similar pattern from person to person. The proviso in the definition 'with no apparent cause other than that of vascular disease' excludes other common causes of damage to the brain such as trauma. The definition does not depend on fancy technology and can be made at the bedside by the doctor. The strict use of this definition has been essential in epidemiological studies assessing stroke incidence and prevalence around the world, and studies of stroke treatment and outcome. However, as time has gone by there have been increasing problems with this formal definition. The most powerful medical treatment for stroke, namely clot-busting medication (thrombolysis) for cerebral infarction, has to be given within a few hours of stroke onset. You cannot wait for 24 hours to be sure this was a stroke! Subarachnoid haemorrhage is officially a subtype of stroke, but the milder forms of this disease present with headache and no focal or global neurological deficit, and thus this definition is not quite right for all subarachnoid haemorrhages.

Transient ischaemic attack

Medical definition of transient ischaemic attack

A transient ischaemic attack (TIA) is a clinical syndrome characterized by an acute loss of focal cerebral or monocular function with symptoms lasting less than 24 hours and which is thought to be due to inadequate cerebral or ocular blood supply as a result of arterial thrombosis or embolism associated with arterial, cardiac or haematological disease (Hankey and Warlow 1994).

TIAs are not just 'mini-strokes'

In simple terms a TIA is merely a 'mini-stroke', one from which you make a full recovery within 24 hours, but closer attention to the wording reveals three important differences.

◆ TIAs are all ischaemic events. Although short-lived attacks can, very rarely, be due to intracerebral haemorrhage, it is reasonable to assume that all TIAs are ischaemic because of the causes mentioned in the definition, such as arterial thrombosis (blood clot), an embolus (thrombosis from upstream in the blood supply), cardiac disease (of which there are a large number of causes), or haematological disease ('sticky' blood).

◆ A TIA differs from a stroke in that the definition includes a list of the possible causes of the ischaemic attack. This implies a need for medical investigation to identify the cause for a specific patient.

◆ TIAs also include symptoms due to disturbed blood supply to the eye (vascular insufficiency). If the blood flow to the eye becomes sluggish or blood clots (emboli) block the blood supply to the retina of the eye, the retina becomes short of blood (ischaemic) and this causes transient blindness in the one eye. Characteristically, patients describe a shutter coming down at the beginning of the attack. These are often short lived (seconds or minutes) and have been given a variety of different names: transient monocular blindness or, more traditionally, amaurosis fugax.

The importance of these TIAs is that they can be a warning of a more serious stroke to come. Curiously, a permanent occlusion of the retinal arterial supply is called a retinal infarct not a stroke! For reasons which are not quite clear, a TIA due to a 'brain attack' carries a higher risk of future stroke than a TIA due to an 'eye attack'.

There has been a great deal of discussion as to whether the current definitions of stroke and TIA are appropriate for the twenty-first century. Modern brain imaging, such as CT scanning and magnetic resonance scanning (see Chapter 5, Figures 5.2 and 5.3), has clearly shown that cerebral TIAs and ischaemic stroke are the same disease, and it is our artificial time limit of 24 hours that separates the two. However, in an ever-changing world the problem of basing a definition just on the results of brain imaging would mean that what was a TIA today may be called a stroke tomorrow! Such changes to the definition would cause major problems in the science of medicine as doctors would not be able to compare like with like over time. This emphasizes the value of the current clinical definitions: the study of stroke and TIA over time will be comparing like with like, no matter what progress is made in identifying the underlying infarcts or ischaemic brain with advanced brain imaging.

There are further advantages of the current definitions. Different conditions tend to mimic short-duration attacks (TIA) rather than longer attacks (stroke), and this can be helpful information for the doctor.

'Brain attack', a new term for TIA and stroke

As we become more successful in reversing the consequences of stroke, time is of the essence. Treatments need to be started within minutes or hours of the TIA/stroke onset for maximal effect. We simply mustn't wait until the 24 hours is up before deciding what to do as 'time is brain'. There is increasing consensus that a new term, **brain attack**, should be used to describe the typical features of TIA and stroke within the first 24 hours. There are many advantages to this approach. First, there will be the inevitable comparison with 'heart attack', and hopefully a similar public response of urgency. The term also clearly identifies the organ at risk, thus improving public understanding. The use of 'brain attack' will also help to motivate an often sluggish medical response in the emergency room and provide a useful hint that the main conditions mimicking stroke are also brain conditions (such as epilepsy, brain tumours, or multiple sclerosis). The key aim of emergency treatments for 'brain attacks' is to reverse all the neurological symptoms as soon as possible, thus resulting in more TIAs and fewer strokes. At 24 hours, reassessment of patients will identify whether the brain attack has led to a permanent stroke or not.

Other definitions and names

A variety of other names and definitions have been proposed over the years.

- **Apoplexy** The ancient term for devastating stroke.

- **Cerebrovascular accident** The term for stroke used in the mid-twentieth century and still enshrined in some medical search engines and registers. It is not a useful medical term nowadays. Stroke is not an accident, and many people use the term CVA in a confusing manner. For example, 'the patient had a right CVA' is alternatively interpreted as a right hemiparesis or a right brain stroke (which would usually cause a left hemiparesis). This term is best abandoned.

- **CITS (cerebral infarction with transient signs)** This was proposed when CT scanning revealed that about a fifth of patients with TIA had definite evidence of new cerebral infarction on brain imaging.

- **RIND (reversible ischaemic neurological deficit)** This has been proposed to describe a stroke that leads to full recovery.

Haemorrhagic stroke

Stroke due to haemorrhage continues to have a variety of different names. The official medical term for haemorrhagic stroke is **primary intracerebral haemorrhage (PICH)**, and the volume of blood in a PICH is often referred to as a **haematoma**, or confusingly as a **blood clot**. Any abnormal blood within the skull is called **intracranial haemorrhage**. Bleeding around the brain may be due to a **subdural haematoma** (but this is not usually called a stroke). **Subarachnoid haemorrhage** may be pure subarachnoid bleeding but may also arise from a **PICH**. Finally, some cerebral infarcts bleed and this is called **haemorrhagic transformation of infarction**.

Further reading

Hankey GJ, Warlow CP (1994) *Transient Ischaemic Attacks of the Brain and Eye.*
    WB Saunders–Baillière Tindall, London.
Hatano S (1976) Experience from a multicentre stroke register: a preliminary report.
    Bulletin of the World Health Organization, **54**, 541–53.

2

How common is stroke?

 Key points

- Stroke is common, with a typical incidence of 1.5–2 people having a stroke per 1000 population each year.

- Stroke is rare in children but becomes increasingly common with increasing age.

- Asia has the largest number of people with strokes in the world.

- The funding for stroke services and research is generally poor compared with the human misery of the condition.

The answer to the question 'How common is stroke?' depends on the context. For example, in 1997 an investigation of the global burden of disease was published (Murray and Lopez 1997), and the authors estimated that in 1990 there were just over 50 million deaths in the world, and stroke was the second most common cause with about 4.5 million deaths annually. The top 10 causes of death are shown in Table 2.1. However, deaths are a crude way of looking at the burden of disease. Stroke **incidence** tells us how many new strokes occur each year, and stroke **prevalence** tells us how many people are alive having survived a stroke.

Stroke incidence

Globally, stroke incidence is staggering, with about 16 million people having a stroke each year. A third of these will die from their stroke (10 per cent of global deaths) and another third will survive with disability. This results in about 62 million stroke survivors globally, about half of whom will be disabled. Clearly, stroke is a common condition.

Table 2.1 The top 10 cause of deaths in 1990

Cause of death	Millions per year worldwide
Ischaemic heart disease	6.3
Stroke	4.4
Lower respiratory infections	4.3
Diarrhoeal diseases	2.9
Perinatal disorders	2.4
Chronic obstructive pulmonary disease	2.2
Tuberculosis (without HIV infection)	2.0
Measles	1.0
Road traffic accidents	0.99
Respiratory cancers	0.94

Adapted from *Lancet* Editorial, **349**, 1263 (1997).

Incidence figures are of great interest as they tell us our chances of having a stroke. Stroke incidence data will also inform decisions on health planning, as they can be used to estimate the resources required in the acute phase (e.g. acute hospital beds). Stroke incidence has been measured in a variety of countries over a number of years and, when corrected for differences in the age and sex mix of these different populations, have produced similar results, with an incidence about 1.5–2 per 1000 population per year. Although it is difficult to obtain an accurate estimate of major differences in stroke incidence around the world, studies have demonstrated a lower stroke rate in France and a much higher rate in the East European states. It is very likely that these rates simply reflect differences in the major vascular risk factors in these populations. The main uncertainty in stroke incidence around the world is in India and China. Each of these countries has a population of over a billion individuals, with great diversity of socio-economic background and vascular risk factors. Incidence studies in one part of China may not be representative of other areas. The rapid change in vascular risk factors also adds to the uncertainty. Nevertheless each of these countries will be shouldering a stroke burden of several million a year. Table 2.2 shows estimates of the total number of strokes likely per year in selected countries around the world. The burden of stroke in Asia is the real global challenge.

Table 2.2 Estimated population incidence of stroke (first and recurrent) in selected countries worldwide

Country	Population (millions)	Number of people having a stroke each year
Argentina	36	106 000
Australia	20	53 000
Austria	8	20 000
Bangladesh	142	192 000
Belgium	10	20 000
Brazil	186	387 000
Bulgaria	8	34 000
Canada	32	50 000
Chile	16	24 000
China	1316	2 500 000*
Czech Republic	10	46 000
Denmark	5	10 000
Egypt	74	100 000
Finland	5	14 000
France	64	140 000
Georgia	4	45 000
Germany	82	180 000
Greece	10	22 000
Hungary	10	51 000
India	1103	1 500 000*
Indonesia	223	300 000
Iran	70	100 000
Iraq	29	24 000
Ireland	4	10 000
Israel	7	15 000

(Continued)

Table 2.2 Estimated population incidence of stroke (first and recurrent) in selected countries worldwide (*continued*)

Country	Population (millions)	Number of people having a stroke each year
Italy	58	165 000
Japan	128	300 000
Kenya	34	42 000
Lithuania	3	15 000
Malaysia	25	30 000
Mexico	107	78 000
Netherlands	16	30 000
New Zealand	4	7000
Nigeria	131	207 000
Norway	5	13 000
Pakistan	160	250 000
Philippines	83	72 000
Poland	39	59 000
Portugal	10	20 000
Romania	22	150 000
Russian Federation	147	323 000
Saudia Arabia	25	9000
Serbia and Montenegro	11	60 000
Singapore	4	3000
Slovakia	5	21 000
Slovenia	2	4000
South Africa	47	90 000
Spain	40	89 000
Sweden	9	30 000

(Continued)

Table 2.2 Estimated population incidence of stroke (first and recurrent) in selected countries worldwide (*continued*)

Country	Population (millions)	Number of people having a stroke each year
Switzerland	8	13 000
Thailand	65	150 000
Turkey	60	78 000
United Arab Emirates	5	1500
UK	60	130 000
USA	298	700 000
Uruguay	3	9000
Venezuala	27	24 000
Vietnam	84	174 000

*The sheer size of the populations of India and China exaggerate the uncertainties of these figures which could be under- or over-estimates by 500 000–1 000 000.

The figures are extrapolated from incidence studies, national stroke associations, and expert opinion or derived from World Health Organization stroke mortality data. Some may be rather inaccurate, but they are based on the best available data.

Hidden around the stroke incident rate of about 1.5–2 per 1000 population per year is the enormous difference in stroke incidence at different ages (Table 2.3). There is a 10-fold increase in stroke incidence from childhood to early adulthood, a further 10-fold increase between early adulthood and middle age, and a further 10-fold increase from middle age to old age. In addition, about half of all childhood strokes occur in the first 28 days of life (the neonatal period) and the rest in later childhood.

In general, stroke incidence figures from medical research papers refer to a 'first-ever' stroke, and a rule of thumb is to increase these incidence figures by about a third to account for all strokes occurring, thus including 'first-ever' and secondary strokes.

Stroke prevalence

The prevalence of stroke is much more difficult to measure, and for that reason is less frequently the subject of medical research. Overall prevalence rates

Table 2.3 Incidence of stroke in different age bands

Age range (years)	Approximate incidence (strokes per 100 000 per year) per age group
All age groups	150–200
Childhood	2
16–44	5–20
45–54	50–100
55–64	200–300
65–74	500–1000
75–84	1000–2000
85+	2000–3000

are probably about 10 per 1000 population, which corresponds to about 50 per 1000 for those over 65 years of age. This figure will vary widely depending on the age distribution of the population, the prevalence of vascular risk factors, and success in acute treatment (stroke units) and stroke secondary prevention. However, prevalence data are very useful for identifying the need for medical services (patients who have survived stroke have a high risk of future vascular disease) and support services (as a third of stroke survivors are left with disability).

Outcome of stroke

As discussed earlier, stroke is an important cause of death. Some strokes are rapidly fatal, particularly primary intracerebral haemorrhage or very large ischaemic strokes, contributing to an early mortality of about 10 per cent within the first week of stroke. A further 10 per cent die within a month, and after about a year a third of people with stroke will have died. As time goes on, the risk of recurrent stroke tends to fall, but the risk of other vascular disease becomes more important and after 10 years 80 per cent of people with stroke will have died – the majority from vascular disease.

Priorities for stroke

Many will be surprised at the facts and figures in this chapter. Stroke is clearly a common problem with substantial human misery arising from the distressingly high fatality rate and resulting disability in survivors. However, stroke is not a high priority for many health services, public charitable donations, or government research funding. Heart disease and cancer are much more generously funded. Perhaps this is because stroke mainly occurs in old age, possibly reflecting some ageism. Given that stroke is largely preventable and we can potentially eliminate the majority of strokes, it is strange that stroke medicine and its prevention is not a higher priority around the world. Imagine the excitement if cancer doctors found a cure for most cancers!

Further reading

Feigin VL, Lawes CMM, Bennett DA, and Anderson CS (2003) Stroke epidemiology: a review of population-based studies of incidence, prevalence, and case-fatality in the 20th century. *Lancet Neurology*, **2**, 43–53.

Murray CJD and Lopez AD (1997) Mortality by cause for eight regions of the world: Global Burden of Disease Study. *Lancet*, **349**, 1269–76.

Pendlebury ST, Rothwell PM, Algra A, *et al.* (2004) Underfunding of stroke research: a Europe-wide problem. *Stroke*, **35**, 2368–71.

World Health Organization websites. http://www.who.int/whosis/mort/profiles/en/index.html and http://www.who.int/en/

3

Who gets strokes?

→ Key points

- The important stroke risk factors are increasing age, male gender, high blood pressure, high blood cholesterol, diabetes, smoking, atrial fibrillation, and excessive alcohol.

- There are numerous other weaker stroke risk factors, but these are responsible for less than 10 per cent of all strokes.

- Many stroke risk factors are reversible or can be treated successfully, and thus most stroke is theoretically preventable.

A simple answer to the question 'Who gets strokes?' is people with diseased heart and blood vessels, damaged by a lifetime of high blood pressure and the build-up of fatty deposits in the bloodstream, and the older you are the more likely you are to have accumulated these problems. The more complex answer is that everyone is at risk, but for some the risks are tiny (e.g. children) and for others the risk is large (e.g. someone with an artificial heart valve).

Risk factors for stroke

Risk factors for stroke are the characteristics (of an individual or population) that are associated with an increased risk of stroke compared with those without those characteristics.

Before we discuss the main risk factors for stroke we need to consider some philosophical problems with this sort of discussion. Although we know the important stroke risk factors, it is often impossible to know which one was to blame for a particular individual's stroke. Some people have many risk factors, any one of which is known to be associated with an increased risk. These risk factors, in isolation or combination, often lead to an identifiable **cause** of stroke. Conversely, some people have no obvious stroke risk factors, but have a stroke because of a definite cause such as carotid dissection due to being hit in the neck, which is a most unfortunate accident. In other people with stroke, the cause is never identified, and medically this is termed **cryptogenic stroke**. The paradox of risk factors is that some risk factors, in population terms, only have a small likelihood of causing stroke, but if you are the unlucky person with a stroke due to this 'weak' risk factor, you are unlikely to consider this a small risk! Epidemiologists try and quantify how many strokes are due to each risk factor with the term **attributable risk**, and wherever possible I will try and put the risk factor in perspective by estimating this attributable risk.

Epidemiology

Epidemiology is the branch of medicine that deals with the incidence, distribution, and control of disease in a population.

Stroke is largely a preventable disease

One of my favourite articles from the medical literature makes an important point: you can find certain populations in the world where stroke is unheard of, and vascular disease is not evident, even on objective testing. Lindeberg and Lundh (1993) travelled to Papua New Guinea and studied the people of Kitava who followed a traditional Melanesian subsistence life. By interview they were unable to find anyone who had previously had a stroke-like episode, nor could these people recall anyone dying of such a syndrome. This wonderful description is a wake-up call for the public – stroke is largely a disease of our times which is due to our current lifestyle.

Most strokes are due to the complications of damage to the blood vessels or the heart, particularly narrowing of the blood vessels due to the build-up of fatty deposits (atheroma) and hardening of the arteries because of high blood pressure. The risk factors for this sort of vascular disease are well known and are (in approximate order of importance) increasing age, high blood pressure, cigarette smoking, diabetes mellitus, and high blood cholesterol. Therefore it follows that these well-known vascular risk factors are also important risk factors for stroke. Increasing age, high blood pressure, and excessive alcohol intake are the main risk factors for primary intracerebral haemorrhage stroke.

Overall, high blood pressure is the most important risk factor for stroke, as it can cause both of the main types of stroke (ischaemic stroke and primary intracerebral haemorrhage).

When epidemiologists are looking for the **cause** of diseases, possible risk factors must satisfy a whole series of criteria before causation is proved. In brief, these rules are as follows:

♦ a consistent association between the risk factor and the disease

♦ a biologically plausible mechanism

♦ a dose–response relationship, i.e. more of the risk factor produces more disease.

♦ a reduction in disease when the risk factor is successfully removed or treated.

When these conditions are met, causation has been proved. In stroke medicine, hypertension, or more accurately high blood pressure, definitely meets these criteria. Raised blood pressure is consistently associated with stroke around the world. Higher blood pressures have been shown to be a more potent cause of stroke than lower pressures, and the abnormal blood vessels associated with raised blood pressure are known to be a cause of stroke (e.g. atheroma of the carotid bulb, hypertensive heart disease causing atrial fibrillation, and ruptured arterioles due to high perfusion pressures). Crucially, randomized controlled trials of blood pressure tablets for people with hypertension (and more recently for those with traditionally 'normal' blood pressures) have been shown to reduce the subsequent risk of stroke.

High blood pressure

The use of the term 'high blood pressure' is deliberate, as older terms such as 'hypertension' are inadequate in describing the association between blood pressure and stroke. Over a surprisingly large range of blood pressure levels, a higher blood pressure is associated with a higher risk of stroke (both ischaemic and haemorrhagic). The evidence suggests that high blood pressure is a more potent risk factor for primary intracerebral haemorrhage. Previously, the term hypertension was used when a certain level of blood pressure was thought to be particularly dangerous and amenable to intervention (lifestyle changes or medication). Historically, the main reason to treat hypertension was to prevent strokes, as the stroke prevention benefit appears within a few months (the benefit in preventing heart disease is smaller and takes many more years of blood pressure treatment). There is no 'magic' threshold at which someone suddenly becomes high risk. In fact, the decision to lower blood pressure

Stroke · the**facts**

is now known to depend on many other factors. A non-smoking woman aged 50 years with a low blood cholesterol and a blood pressure of 135/80 mmHg (see box) does not need medication to lower blood pressure, but a 50-year-old diabetic man who smokes cigarettes with a similar blood pressure would benefit from a lower blood pressure. In general, adults should ensure that their usual blood pressure is below 140/85 mmHg, but the treatment threshold will differ depending on other risk factors. High blood pressure is the most important modifiable risk factor for stroke, and epidemiologists have estimated that this one factor alone is responsible for probably about half of all strokes. Preventative methods will be described in Chapter 8.

Blood pressure measurement

Blood pressure is measured with a sphygmomanometer. An inflatable cuff is placed on the upper arm and the inflated until the pulse at the wrist disappears. The cuff is then deflated slowly whilst the observer listens to the sounds of the blood in the artery at the elbow. Two numbers are recorded, called systolic and diastolic blood pressures, and the units (millimetres of mercury) reflect the fact mercury was used in the older sphygmomanometers to measure these pressures. Mercury is highly toxic, and so most modern machines are aneroid or electronic. However, the units are still millimetres of mercury (mmHg).

We obviously need our blood pressure to be sufficient to perfuse the brain and other vital organs, but it is likely that lifelong blood pressures below 100/70 mmHg were normal in societies without vascular disease. All of us will feel faint and lose consciousness if our blood pressure falls too low (e.g. a simple faint on a hot day), and this threshold level of blood pressure will vary from person to person. Many people have troublesome symptoms associated with low blood pressure due to medication, older age, or disease, and so a careful balance must be sought. If blood pressure is too high, the risks of stroke become important. If blood pressure is too low, troublesome fainting (syncopal attacks) will occur. It can be difficult to get the balance right in some people. (In my department I put people on antihypertensive medication in the stroke clinic, and my colleague takes people off similar medication in the syncope clinic. The trick is to make sure that not many patients have to attend both clinics!) Current epidemiology suggests that our Western lifestyles have moved too far towards the 'high' blood pressure range, and we need to try and alter our habits if we want to have a lower risk of stroke. It is interesting to speculate why only some people with high blood pressure get strokes, and researchers

22

have wondered about possible causal mechanisms. Perhaps some people have surges of particularly high blood pressure which cause a stroke there and then (see patient's perspective below).

Ways in which blood pressure can be treated will be discussed in Chapter 8.

 Case study

Sudden bad news

An elderly man was informed that his wife had just died. She had been expected to die from her illness for some time. He went to the bathroom and collapsed. An ambulance was summoned and he was taken to hospital. In hospital a CT scan showed a large primary intracerebral haemorrhage and unfortunately he died a few days later. His family gave permission for a post-mortem examination which showed acute fibrinoid necrosis (cell death) of the small blood vessels of the brain. What had caused his stroke? Was it a sudden surge of blood pressure after he had been given bad news? Is this the explanation for the actual reason some people with hypertensive disease have a stroke?

Cigarette smoking

Most people are aware of the risks of smoking, but few are aware of how risky it is. Sir Richard Doll's famous study of smoking by UK male doctors (Fig. 3.1) emphasized these risks with some simple statistics. The evidence from the remarkable 50-year follow-up of these doctors illustrated that smokers died on average 10 years prematurely, and that about half of all smokers would die prematurely as a result of their habit. These risks are enormous when compared with the many other things people worry about. The good news is that on stopping smoking you can halve your future vascular risk (and this includes stroke). Cigarette smoking is probably responsible for about 15 per cent of all strokes in the UK, but will be a more important cause in countries with greater smoking prevalence.

Atrial fibrillation

Atrial fibrillation (AF) is the name given to the irregular and uncoordinated beating of the heart. It has three main consequences: the heart often beats too fast, causing palpitation and a drop in blood pressure; the heart becomes less efficient as a 'pump' and this can lead to heart failure; and the condition is

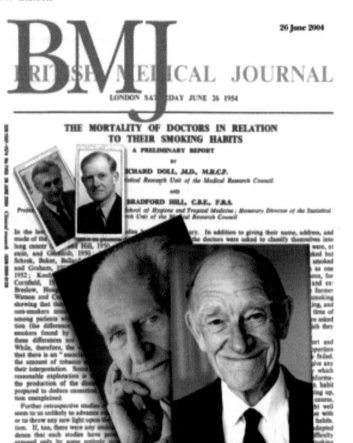

Figure 3.1 The 50-year follow-up of the famous study of British doctors by Richard Doll and colleagues (which identified the dangers of smoking), together with a reproduction of the original publication, was published in the *British Medical Journal*, 26 June 2004. Cover image reproduced with permission.

Table 3.1 Causes of atrial fibrillation

Cardiac disease	Non-cardiac disease
Ischaemic heart disease (including acute myocardial infarction (heart attack)*)	Over-active thyroid (thyrotoxicosis)*
Hypertension	Pneumonia*
Rheumatic heart disease	Infection*
Cardiac surgery or catheterization	Electrolyte abnormalities*
Sick sinus syndrome	Cancer
Cardiomyopathy	Clots in the lung (pulmonary embolism)*
Pericardial disease	
Congenital heart disease	
Atrial septal defect	
Atrial myxoma	

*AF is often short-lived if the underlying problem is treated.

associated with formation of blood clots in the heart (usually the left atrium). This fast uncoordinated heart rhythm occasionally causes blood clots to be pumped out of the heart into the circulation, and a stroke occurs if these become lodged in the blood supply to the brain. The prevalence of atrial fibrillation increases with age and is associated with many medical conditions (Table 3.1). In early middle age (50–59 years old) about 1 in 200 people have AF, and this prevalence approximately doubles each decade to about 10 per cent at age 80–89 years. AF in children and young adults is usually associated with heart disease (Table 3.1).

Because AF occasionally causes blood clots to form in the heart, people with AF have a fivefold risk of stroke compared with those who do not have AF. Because of the rapid increase in the prevalence of this abnormality with age, the proportion of strokes due to AF rises from 1–2 per cent at age 50–59 years to about 20 per cent in those aged 80 years and older. Overall, AF probably causes about 10 per cent of all strokes in a country like the UK. However, as about a fifth of all stroke patients have AF at the time of their stroke, about half of these strokes are not due to AF.

Diabetes mellitus

Diabetes mellitus is a very important risk factor for stroke because of two main factors: it is increasingly common, and it is an independent risk factor for ischaemic stroke (approximately doubling the risk). There are now nearly 2 million diabetics in the UK, an increase of 500 000 in the past decade. In the USA, the prevalence of type 2 diabetes has doubled from 4 to 8 per cent in the past 40 years, in China the prevalence in adults has tripled from 1 to 3.2 per cent between 1980 and 1996, and elsewhere in Asia the increase is even more alarming with rates increasing three-to fivefold in countries such as Thailand and Indonesia in the past 30 years. Diabetics usually have higher blood pressures and higher blood cholesterol levels, and so are at particularly high risk of vascular disease. Studies adjusting for these other risk factors still found that the presence of diabetes doubled the risk of stroke. Therefore the rapid rise in obesity, and thus in type 2 diabetes, will increase the risk of stroke from this cause. Diabetes (or raised blood glucose levels) probably causes 10–20 per cent of all strokes.

Cholesterol

Cholesterol is an essential component of the body as it makes up part of the cell wall and is also required to make hormones and bile acids. Most cholesterol is actually manufactured by the body (usually in the liver) rather than obtained from the diet, but an increase in saturated fat consumption leads to an increase in blood cholesterol. Blood cholesterol is transported in the blood by 'protein suitcases' called lipoproteins, as cholesterol itself is insoluble in blood. Low-density lipoprotein (LDL-cholesterol) carries cholesterol from the liver to the tissues, and it is this type of cholesterol that is associated with ischaemic stroke and heart disease. High-density lipoprotein (HDL-cholesterol) carries cholesterol from the tissues to the liver, and increased levels of HDL seem to protect against vascular disease. Hence LDL-cholesterol is bad cholesterol, and HDL-cholesterol is good cholesterol.

A particular enzyme, called HMG-Co A reductase, increases the production of cholesterol in the body, and medication to inhibit this enzyme (the statins) has been proved to dramatically reduce blood LDL-cholesterol with a corresponding decrease in heart attacks and ischaemic stroke (see Chapter 8).

Few foods contain cholesterol; eggs, liver, kidney, and prawns are some examples of cholesterol-laden food. However, diets high in saturated fats (such as the fats in butter, lard, and hard cheese) lead to elevated LDL-cholesterol levels. Monosaturated fats (such as the fats in olive oil and avocado) and polyunsaturated fats (such as fats in sunflower oil and fish oil) are better for your health. In addition, exercise can increase HDL-cholesterol, which is one explanation of why exercise is good for you.

The association between cholesterol and stroke has been difficult to sort out because there are three very different types of stroke (ischaemic stroke, primary intracerebral haemorrhage, and subarachnoid haemorrhage). Cholesterol appears to have different effects on ischaemic stroke than on haemorrhagic stroke, with high blood cholesterol being a risk factor for ischaemic stroke and low blood cholesterol possibly being a risk factor for haemorrhagic stroke. The previous confusion about whether cholesterol was a risk factor for stroke arose because the older epidemiological studies did not identify the type of stroke and thus the effect of blood cholesterol levels on ischaemic stroke was obscured. The reason we are now confident that cholesterol is a risk factor for ischaemic stroke is that trials of cholesterol-lowering medication have reduced the subsequent risk of ischaemic stroke. High cholesterol probably causes about 5–10 per cent of all strokes.

The epidemiological association between low blood cholesterol levels and haemorrhagic stroke is intriguing and remains controversial. A recent study has suggested that this association may be explained by high alcohol intake and high blood pressure, and thus low blood cholesterol may not be associated with haemorrhagic stroke at all. Of note, in two of the largest randomized controlled trials of cholesterol lowering for people with stroke disease, there was a small increase in haemorrhagic stroke in those allocated cholesterol-lowering therapy. A further explanation is that high blood pressure and low blood cholesterol make haemorrhagic stroke more likely, and high blood pressure and high blood cholesterol make ischaemic strokes more likely.

The risk factors of increasing age, high blood pressure, high blood cholesterol, cigarette smoking, atrial fibrillation, and diabetes can be considered the core risk factors for ischaemic stroke, and other known risk factors may exert their effect through these factors. For example, the excess stroke risk of obesity may be wholly explained by the increased blood pressure, blood cholesterol, and diabetes seen in obese people (metabolic syndrome). Similarly, if these vascular risk factors have already caused symptoms due to atheromatous disease elsewhere, patients are at higher risk of stroke (Fig. 3.2). Other risk factors such as fibrinogen, may simply reflect the biological mechanisms of the results of the vascular risk factors on the subsequent risk of stroke (e.g. smoking increases fibrinogen levels).

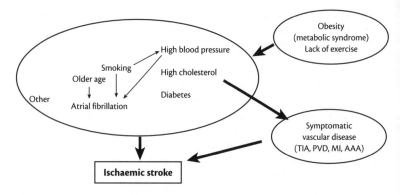

Figure 3.2 Some of the interactions between risk factors for ischaemic stroke: TIA, transient ischaemic attack; AAA, abdominal aortic aneurysm; PVD, peripheral vascular disease; MI, myocardial infarction.

Symptomatic vascular disease

Patients who already have symptomatic vascular disease are at increased risk of stroke compared with age- and sex-matched populations. For example, people with a TIA have a risk of stroke about 10 times that of people without TIA. People with peripheral vascular disease, recent myocardial infarction, previous stroke, or known abdominal aortic aneurysm are similarly at a higher risk of stroke. Symptomatic atheroma in one part of the body predicts similar atheroma in the blood supply to the brain, in particular the aortic arch, the carotid bifurcation, and the vertebral arteries. People with any of these vascular diseases should make efforts to reduce their vascular risk factors to reduce their risk of heart attack and stroke.

Carotid stenosis

Atheroma characteristically forms in the blood vessels in the neck leading to the brain, particularly where the carotid artery divides into two branches. If this blood vessel is narrowed, you can sometimes hear a whooshing noise (bruit) with a stethoscope placed on the neck. As this area is easy to examine, listening for bruits or investigating the narrowing with carotid ultrasound has been feasible for many years. It has been known for many decades that narrowing of the carotid artery (stenosis) is a risk factor for stroke, but it was only when the results of randomized controlled trials of the effect of removing this narrowing were published that the importance of this risk became apparent. This operation is called a carotid endarterectomy, and involves removing the narrowed atheromatous plaque lining the carotid artery. If people have had a TIA or stroke which, after tests, has been shown to be due to a tight carotid stenosis, most of the subsequent strokes for these people are also due to the same problem, i.e. the stenosis is the cause of stroke. If you have carotid stenosis, your risk of stroke depends on many factors. A recent TIA or minor ischaemic stroke in that vascular territory puts you at very high risk. If you have a carotid stenosis but have never had a stroke or TIA, you have a risk of stroke that is probably about two to three times that of someone without a stenosis, which equates to an annual risk of about 1 in 50 (or 2 per cent). This is called asymptomatic stenosis. Another important point to be made about people with carotid disease is that it is a sign of generalized atheroma with subsequent higher risk of heart attacks or vascular disease elsewhere.

Obesity

Studies have demonstrated that stroke is associated with increasing obesity. However, it is uncertain whether obesity is an 'independent' risk factor as this increased risk is mainly due to the common medical problems accompanying obesity, namely high blood pressure, diabetes, and high blood cholesterol (Fig. 3.2). Studies in this area are complicated by the fact that cigarette smoking is associated with thinner people, but smoking itself carries a substantial risk for stroke. A recent large study from Scotland with about 15 000 participants confirmed that obesity was associated with stroke, but when analyses were adjusted for the common vascular risk factors, the association was only just positive and not statistically significant. Overall, there is no doubt that obesity is bad for your vascular health, but this is mainly explained by the consequences of the **metabolic syndrome** of high blood cholesterol, high blood pressure, and diabetes. Obesity may still be an independent risk factor stroke but, if so, it is only a weak risk factor. Another reason that we do not have strong evidence linking obesity to stroke as an independent risk factor is that there are no intervention trials that have studied the success of weight loss in reducing stroke. These trials are very difficult to perform, but studies have shown that weight loss can reduce blood pressure, suggesting that such strategies should achieve an eventual reduction in stroke.

Lack of exercise

The issue of exercise is similar to that of obesity. Regular exercise of sufficient exertion to work up a sweat has major benefits for your vascular health by lowering blood pressure, increasing HDL cholesterol, and preventing diabetes. The benefit of exercise is probably entirely explained by the benefits on these potent stroke risk factors.

Table 3.2 Some rarer causes of stroke

Pregnancy
Race
Psychological stress
'Sticky blood' (numerous possible causes)
Inherited causes
Oral contraceptive pill
Migraine
Obstructive sleep apnoea

The above common risk factors account for the majority of strokes but there are numerous other risk factors that have been associated with stroke (see Table 3.2). Some of the more interesting ones are discussed below.

Alcohol

The epidemiology of alcohol and stroke is interesting and rather complicated. The epidemiology suggests that moderate alcohol, i.e. within the usual recommended daily limits (see box), does not increase the risk of stroke; indeed, many observational studies have shown that moderate alcohol consumption is associated with a lower risk of stroke than that of abstainers. However, we need to be cautious as epidemiological studies can be confounded by other factors. For example, the sort of people who drink moderately ('sensibly') may be the sort of people who do other sensible things with their lives, and it may be these other factors which confer the lower risk of stroke. This is almost certainly what happened in the hormone replacement therapy story (see later). The second reason to be cautious is that alcohol can increase blood pressure, and there is no doubt that a higher blood pressure will lead to a higher risk of stroke. The third reason to be cautious is that heavy or excessive drinking is definitely a risk factor for stroke, perhaps more so for primary intracerebral haemorrhage than for ischaemic stroke. The final reason to be cautious about alcohol is the population approach. The epidemiologist Geoffrey Rose made the point that with a factor like alcohol consumption (or blood pressure, or happiness), the population average predicted the number of 'deviants'. In other words, the promotion of 'moderate' alcohol intake in the general population is likely to increase the number of people drinking dangerously excessively. Similarly, the mean population blood pressure predicts the number of hypertensives, the mean happiness levels predict the number of people with depression, etc. Hence a public health conundrum: promote moderate alcohol consumption for vascular health, and you risk increasing problem alcohol consumption (and move people from the stroke clinic to the liver clinic). My practical advice to patients regarding cigarettes and alcohol is to stop smoking and not to worry too much about the alcohol (unless it is particularly excessive). As a house officer on a liver unit I was always impressed how clean the arteries looked at post-mortem examination. Clearly, the patient and the liver were not so well!

Example of recommended alcohol limits

The Australian National Health and Medical Research Council (NH&MRC) has provided guidelines for safe daily drinking limits. *The recommended maximum for men is four standard drinks per day. For women it is two standard drinks per day. One standard drink contains 10 grams of alcohol,* and is equivalent to one ordinary beer (half a pint), a small glass of wine (100 ml), or a nip of spirits (30 ml).

Fibrinogen

Fibrinogen is a protein that can be measured in the blood, and it is clearly associated with a higher risk of vascular disease. However, it is also clearly associated with other strong risk factors such as smoking, and so it is more of general interest than of practical use.

Recreational drug use

Recreational drugs are illegal in most countries, with alcohol and cigarettes being the common exceptions to this rule. There are a large number of such agents, and no doubt more will appear as human ingenuity continues apace. Sadly, all these drugs (like their legal medical counterparts) have side effects and some have been strongly linked to stroke. Perhaps the most potent is cocaine, and the mechanism for this is thought to be its effect on increasing blood pressure, causing vasospasm or perhaps altering platelet function. Haemorrhagic strokes due to illicit drugs can be a particular problem in younger people, and a drug screen is now an important investigation for younger people with stroke. One report has suggested that cocaine-induced haemorrhagic stroke may be related to underlying vascular problems such as aneurysms or arteriovenous malformations, and the drug use has merely brought these abnormalities to light.

Ecstasy can sometimes cause venous sinus thrombosis (blood clots in the veins that drain the blood from the brain) and cause a stroke.

 Case study

Ecstasy party

A 22-year-old girl enjoyed an all-night rave party during which she took ecstasy tablets. The following day she developed a severe headache which did not improve despite some simple analgesia. Two days after the party she started getting a migrainous aura of flashing lights and holes in her vision. She was admitted to hospital and her examination was essentially normal, as was a CT scan, but her headaches continued. A lumbar puncture was abnormal with a high protein count. The following day she developed some arm weakness, and a further CT scan showed a stroke with evidence of venous sinus thrombosis. She was given heparin to break up the blood clots (anticoagulation) and made a full recovery.

Gender

Men have a higher risk of stroke than women, but interestingly this excess appears greatest at ages around 45–65 years. As stroke risk increases with age and women live longer than men, overall more women have strokes than men.

Strokes as a result of medical management or treatment

Illness due to medical intervention is known as iatrogenic disease, and it is a fact of life that strokes can complicate some treatments. There are some well-known causes – most people are aware that stroke can complicate a surgical operation. Some procedures have a high risk of stroke; for example, cardiac surgery with heart bypass is associated with about a 1–2 per cent risk of stroke and a 30–50 per cent risk of asymptomatic cerebral infarcts if brain scanning (e.g. with advanced magnetic resonance imaging (MRI)) is used to screen for silent strokes after the operation.

Other risks are less obvious, and their detection requires surprisingly large studies. One important example is the issue of hormone replacement therapy (HRT). By the early 1990s a large number of observational studies had shown an association between HRT use and a lower risk of vascular disease in women. Although this observation came from observational epidemiology (rather than the more methodologically vigorous randomized controlled trial), many experts started to recommend HRT as a 'vascular protective' pill. Therefore the medical community was rather shocked when the results of the Women's Health Initiative trial were published in 2002 and showed that HRT for older women was not only ineffective as vascular disease prevention but was actually significantly associated with an excess of coronary heart disease and stroke. Indeed, it has been calculated that, at its peak, HRT probably caused an excess of 6000 strokes per year in the USA. This was not spotted prior to the trial because the actual individual risk is extremely low (but real). This provides a very important lesson. If millions of people take a pill which has a tiny but real risk of stroke, the end result for the population can be thousands of extra strokes. A similar problem was seen with the popular arthritis pill rofecoxib and heart attacks. Observational epidemiology is often not reliable enough to detect these small but important risks, which usually require very large randomized controlled trials to detect uncommon but important side effects. New medications to watch out for include any treatments that could increase blood pressure (or increase blood cholesterol or blood glucose) as these are very likely to increase the risk of stroke.

Strokes in young adults and children will be dealt with in the next chapter.

Further reading

Doll R, Peto R, Boreham J, and Sutherland I (2004). Mortality in relation to smoking: 50 years' observations on male British doctors. *British Medical Journal*, **328**, 1519.

Goldberg IJ, Mosca L, Piano MR, and Fisher EA (2001) Wine and your heart: a science advisory for healthcare professionals from the Nutrition Committee, Council of Epidemiology and Prevention, and Council on Cardiovascular Nursing of the American Heart Association. *Stroke*, **32**, 591–4.

Lammie GA, Lindley R, Keir S, and Wiggam I (2000) Stress-related primary intracerebral hemorrhage: autopsy clues to underlying mechanism. *Stroke*, **31**, 1426–8.

Lindeberg S and Lundh R (1993) Apparent absence of stroke and ischaemic heart disease in a traditional Melanesian island: a clinical study in Kitava. *Journal of Internal Medicine*, **233**, 269–75.

MacMahon S, Peto R, Cutler JA, *et al.* (1990) Blood pressure, stroke and coronary heart disease. Part 1: Effects of prolonger differences in blood pressure – evidence from nine prospective observational studies corrected for the regression dilution bias. *Lancet*, **335**, 765–74.

Rose G and Day S (1990) The population mean predicts the number of deviant individuals. *British Medical Journal*, **301**, 1031–4.

Royal College of Physicians (2006) *Atrial Fibrillation: National Clinical Guideline for Management in Primary and Secondary Care*. Lavenham Press, Sudbury, Suffolk. Available online at: http://www.rcplondon.ac.uk/pubs/brochure.aspx?e=33

Shinton R (1997) Lifelong exposures and the potential for stroke prevention: the contribution of cigarette smoking, exercise and body fat. *Journal of Epidemiology and Community Health*, **51**, 138–43.

Stegmayr B and Asplund K (1995) Diabetes as a risk factor for stroke: a population perspective. *Diabetologia*, **38**, 1061–8.

4

The causes of stroke

➡ Key points

◆ Stroke occurs when blood vessels supplying parts of the brain become blocked (ischaemic stroke) or when they rupture (haemorrhagic stroke).

◆ Ischaemic stroke is mainly due to large-vessel disease, small-vessel disease, and cardio-embolic mechanisms.

◆ Haemorrhagic stroke is mainly due to weakened or diseased blood vessels, blood clotting abnormalities, or extremely high blood pressure.

◆ There are many other causes of stroke, but these are rare and more often affect younger adults or children.

In discussing the causes of stroke it is useful to consider ischaemic stroke and primary intracerebral haemorrhage separately. Ischaemic stroke is divided into large-vessel disease (atheroma), cardio-embolic disease, small-vessel disease, iatrogenic disease (stroke as a consequence or side effect of medical treatment or management), and other. Stroke in children and young adults is discussed at the end of the chapter.

Ischaemic stroke

Large-vessel disease

About half of all ischaemic stroke are due to large-vessel disease. Large-vessel disease stroke is caused by the complications of narrowing and occlusion of blood vessels damaged by atheroma, which is the build-up of abnormal arterial wall material predominantly as a result of hypertension, smoking, diabetes, and raised blood cholesterol. Atheroma tends to accumulate in particular parts of the circulation, presumably because of the flow dynamics of blood and the shear stresses on the vessel wall (see Fig. 4.1). The sites relevant for stroke are those on the route from the heart to the brain: the arch of the aorta, the carotid bifurcation, and the carotid syphon (see Fig. 4.1). For reasons that are not well understood, carotid bifurcation atheroma (carotid stenosis) appears to be more common in white Western populations, but narrowing of the internal carotid artery higher up within the skull (carotid syphon) is more common in Asian populations.

Carotid stenosis is the most important **large-vessel disease** as randomized controlled trials (RCTs) have shown that removal of the abnormal atheroma (carotid endarterectomy) can successfully reduce the subsequent risk of stroke for carefully selected people (see Chapter 8). In addition, procedures that open up the narrowed blood vessel wall (e.g. carotid stenting) are also effective, but probably not as effective as carotid endarterectomy. Many were surprised by the effectiveness of a carotid endarterectomy: the RCTs clearly demonstrated that with successful surgery the risk of a stroke arising in that arterial territory was virtually eliminated, thus confirming that most of the subsequent strokes in that territory in patients with symptomatic carotid stenosis (e.g. patients with a recent TIA or minor event in that arterial territory) are due to the carotid stenosis. This is a nice example of an RCT providing important pathophysiological information (carotid stenosis *is* the cause of subsequent strokes in such patients) as well as answering the original RCT question (*is* carotid endarterectomy a successful operation?).

Carotid syphon disease is an important cause of large-vessel stroke, particularly in Asian populations. We are unsure why certain ethnic groups get troublesome atheroma in the neck (extracranial carotid atheroma in white populations) and others get a similar disease within the skull (intracranial carotid syphon stenosis in Chinese populations). It may be due to a differential effect of hypertension and cholesterol; for example, a lower blood cholesterol and higher blood pressure causes intracranial stenosis, and a higher cholesterol and somewhat lower blood pressure causes extracranial stenosis. Carotid disease within the skull is in a much more inaccessible site and currently we do not have proven surgical interventions for this disease (an RCT of stenting/angioplasty is planned in this area).

The other major cause of large-vessel stroke disease is aortic atheromatous disease. Post-mortem and ultrasound studies (transoesophageal echocardiography) have shown that atheroma of the major vessels emerging from the heart is an important cause of stroke. Surgical intervention is not feasible for the majority of patients with this type of disease, and thus lowering of blood pressure

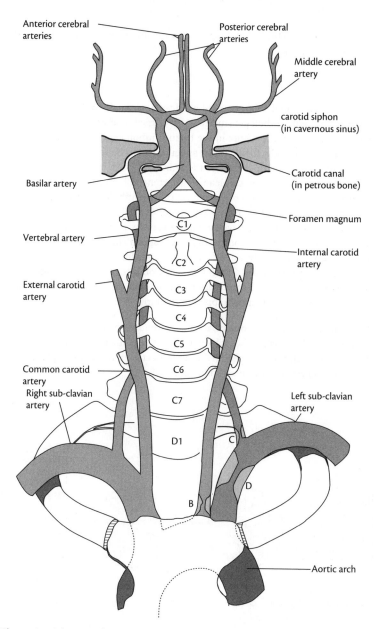

Figure 4.1 Atheroma characteristically develops at key points of stress (A → D) in the blood vessels to the brain as shown here.

and cholesterol and blood-thinning medication are the key preventative strategies for these patients.

Cardio-embolic disease

Emboli are abnormal solid, or semi-solid, materials which flow in the blood stream. Eventually emboli get stuck and block the blood vessels, and this causes ischaemic stroke if it occurs in the brain. Emboli can also cause trouble in other areas of the body: for example, an embolus in the renal artery can cause a renal infarction (death of part of the kidney) and an embolus flowing into the major artery of the leg can lead to gangrene. Obviously these emboli are abnormal and cause serious problems. As cardio-emboli cause about a fifth of ischaemic strokes (see Fig. 4.2), a key aspect of stroke evaluation is to search for this possibility. Table 4.1 lists common sources of emboli. Emboli cannot flow in the bloodstream for long as they are trapped either in the lung or in the arterial supply of the body. For example, a blood clot arising from a thrombosis in the calf muscle veins (a deep venous thrombosis) will, if dislodged, flow to the large veins of the body cavity (inferior vena cava), then into the right side of the heart, and then be trapped in the lung.

By far the most common potential cause of emboli in the brain is the heart condition atrial fibrillation (see Chapter 3). As this is such a common condition, the prevention and treatment of AF is an important part of stroke prevention. The causes of AF are summarized in Table 3.1.

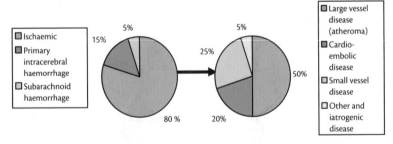

Figure 4.2 Pie charts illustrating (a) the underlying pathology of stroke and (b) the main causes of ischaemic stroke.

Table 4.1 Sources of emboli causing stroke

Thrombotic causes
Atrial fibrillation
Recent heart attack (myocardial infarction)
Poor left ventricular dysfunction
Valvular heart disease
Mechanical heart valves
Infective causes
Infective endocarditis
Infected endoluminal grafts
Syphilis
Paradoxical emboli
Deep vein thrombosis
Other causes
Trauma (cholesterol and air emboli)
Left atrial myxoma
Cardiac surgery
Tumours (cardiac or cancer elsewhere)

Small-vessel disease

Small-vessel disease causes about a quarter of all ischaemic strokes and is also a common cause of primary intracerebral haemorrhage (see below). These small blood vessels can either block or burst. Unfortunately, although these blood vessels only supply a small volume of brain, a stroke due to small-vessel disease can be severe if it occurs in particular parts of the brain, especially parts where many nerve fibres come together. This aspect of stroke disease has been particularly hard to study for several reasons: small-vessel strokes are rarely fatal and thus post-mortem tissue is not available for study; on the rare occasions when pathological material is available, it is incredibly difficult to study these small blood vessels; until very recently brain imaging has been too insensitive to visualize these vessels. As a consequence of this dearth of research, we are uncertain of the cause of many small-vessel disease strokes. Small-vessel occlusion may be caused by any of the following:

◆ very small deposits of atheroma in small blood vessels or where these small vessels branch off from larger vessels (micro-atheroma)

◆ thickening of the small blood vessels as a result of hyaline thickening (arteriolosclerosis)

◆ a more complex thickening called lipohyalinosis or fibrinoid necrosis

◆ the vessels becoming leaky, so that there is too much fluid in the surrounding brain tissue.

Whatever the cause, small-vessel ischaemic stroke disease occurs because of the lack of a good alternative (collateral) blood flow in particular areas of the brain. Thus even one crucially placed blockage will result in part of the brain dying – the cause of cerebral ischaemia and infarction.

Primary intracerebral haemorrhage

There are numerous causes of primary intracerebral haemorrhage, often referred to as **haemorrhagic stroke**. Haemorrhagic stroke is caused by three main mechanisms: the blood vessels are weakened or damaged, the blood is too 'thin' because of a lack of blood clotting factors, or blood pressure becomes too high. Conditions which weaken blood vessels include small-vessel disease, amyloid angiopathy (a condition usually affecting older people or a genetic defect in some families), and vessel abnormalities including cerebral aneurysms, vascular malformations, inflammation of the blood vessels (vasculitis), and trauma. A bleeding tendency (blood too 'thin') may be due to medication such as warfarin (see Chapter 8), or haematological abnormalities such as haemophilia or leukaemia, or thrombolysis treatment (see Chapter 5). High blood pressure is the main risk factor for haemorrhagic stroke as hypertension probably drives the changes that weaken the blood vessels. However, on rare occasions, situations where the blood pressure shoots up, such as acute severe stress, sexual intercourse, and illicit drugs such as amphetamines and cocaine, can also lead to haemorrhagic stroke.

Other causes

There are many other causes of stroke (apart from large-and small-vessel disease, cardio-emboli, and haemorrhage), in fact too many to discuss in a book of this size. This large number of other causes of stroke make up the final 5–10 per cent of stroke. Suffice it to say that any condition, injury, or disease that blocks or damages the blood vessels leading to the brain will cause stroke. Some of these are listed in Table 4.2. A few of these conditions are worth some additional explanation. Sometimes, because of genetic factors or external injury, a blood vessel wall splits internally (a process called **dissection**) and a second lumen forms within the blood vessel. This 'false lumen' can then

Table 4.2 Other causes of stroke

Dissection
Infection
Side effects of medication
Side effects of illicit drugs (e.g. cocaine)
Thrombophilia (genetic increased tendency to form blood clots)
Trauma
Vasculitis

compress the original lumen, blocking the flow of blood and causing a stroke. Interestingly, a dissection of the carotid artery can occasionally have no symptoms at all, yet in other people a similar injury causes a devastating stroke. The range of symptoms from the same problem is characteristic of stroke disease and is due to collateral blood vessels. In some people the collateral circulation is so well developed that the blockage of one (or more) of the major vessels to the brain does not result in any brain injury. Blunt injury to the neck can cause a carotid dissection and, as patients will not be aware of the connection, it is important to ask if this occurred prior to a stroke, particularly if the person has few (or no) classical stroke risk factors.

Infections can occasionally cause stroke, classically syphilis but also infections such as HIV and varicella (chickenpox). Although they are rare, it is important to identify infectious causes as treatment of stroke in these cases should also include treatment of the infection. Many stroke physicians have stopped routinely screening for evidence of syphilis infection, but two recent cases in a hospital near mine last year are a reminder that this can still occur.

Inflammation of blood vessels is also an important cause of stroke and this includes conditions such as the vasculitides (e.g. cranial arteritis).

 Case study

A 75-year-old woman complained of increasing headache and hazy eyesight which her GP attributed to the stress of dealing with her daughter's recent marriage break-up. Two weeks later she developed a stroke. Investigations in hospital showed a very high erythrocyte sedimentation rate (ESR) of 110 mm/hour which strongly suggested cranial arteritis. She was treated with high-dose steroids and her headaches resolved over-night; however, she remained disabled from her stroke.

Lesson: Cranial arteritis should always be excluded if an elderly patient complains of new or continuing headache as steroids can dramatically reduce the risk of stroke or blindness.

Inherited causes

The inherited forms of stroke are all rare. The best known is CADASIL (cerebral autosomal dominant arteriopathy with subcortical infarcts and leuco-encephalopathy) which is, as the name tells us, an autosomal dominantly inherited condition. A careful family history will identify successive generations affected with multiple small-vessel type strokes. Interestingly, in about two out of five cases, the strokes are preceded by migraine. Unfortunately, the accumulation of strokes leads to a progressive increase in disability, with walking particularly affected, and dementia is common.

Strokes in children

As stroke is characteristically a disease of old age, many are surprised to hear that children can be affected. Childhood stroke is rare, with an incidence of 2 per 100 000 children per year (see Table 2.3). Stroke in old age is nearly always due to the complications of atheroma and life-long hypertension; conversely, virtually all childhood stroke is due to other mechanisms. The important childhood causes are the myriad of rare diseases that cause arterial abnormalities such as moya-moya disease, and arteritis, or complications of infection such as meningitis (rare in developed countries) and varicella. Serious illness in childhood, such as infection in premature babies, congenital heart disease, malignancies such as leukaemia, and conditions that thicken the blood (prothrombotic states), are the other important causes. Hidden behind the low childhood incidence rate is an age split; about half of the strokes are seen in neonates and half in later childhood, and this divide is also reflected in the causes of childhood stroke (see Table 4.3). Sickle cell disease is an important cause of childhood stroke in black children as they have a risk of stroke some 200–400 times greater than those without this condition. Most children affected are homozygous for sickle cell disease, and without treatment up to a fifth of such children will have a stroke by the time they reach adulthood. Haemorrhagic stroke in children can be caused by arteriovenous

Table 4.3 Causes of stroke in children

Neonates	Later childhood
75% Idiopathic (unknown)	25% Vasculopathy
5% Vasculopathy	25% Infection
5% Infection	25% Idiopathic
5% Prothrombotic	15% Cardiac
5% Cardiac	10% Prothrombotic
5% Genetic*	

* Sickle cell disease is an important common cause of stroke in black populations.

malformations in the brain, malignancy, trauma, and medical treatment (e.g. warfarin).

Another important difference between childhood stroke and adult stroke is the presenting symptoms. In children, seizures and subtle neurological signs are common. In view of the rather non-specific presentations of stroke, diagnosis can be confused with many other conditions (there are many stroke mimics), and children often present late to medical attention. Studies have demonstrated that after about the age of 15, the causes of stroke are similar to those for young adults (<60 years old).

Strokes in young adults (16–60 years)

In some respects young adults represent a transitional group who have yet to develop serious atheroma or have serious complications of life-long hypertension (the common cause of stroke in old age) but have moved away from the unique risks of neonate life. Therefore stroke in this age group is sometimes due to premature 'usual' vascular disease, but more often than not it is due to rarer problems such as heart abnormalities, genetic predisposition to 'thick blood' (the thrombophilias), and a collection of rare disorders that affect the cranial and extracranial blood vessels. Thus investigation of stroke in this age group involves very detailed examination of the heart and blood vessels looking, for example, for a 'hole in the heart' or a carotid dissection (see above), blood tests to exclude the thrombophilia group of disorders (conditions that lead to sticky blood), exclusion of infection such a syphilis or HIV, medication (e.g. the contraceptive pill), street drugs (e.g. cocaine), or genetic conditions such as mitochondrial disease or CADASIL.

Stroke in pregnancy

The risks of having a stroke whilst pregnant is very low, but is about 13 times greater than that in non-pregnant women of the same age. In practical terms this means that about 1 in 3000 pregnancies will be complicated by a stroke. Some of these strokes are directly caused by the pregnancy (e.g. amniotic fluid embolism), but the majority are due to known causes of stroke exacerbated by the pregnancy such as high blood pressure causing haemorrhage, 'sticky blood', dissection of arteries, heart conditions, and venous sinus thrombosis.

Venous sinus thrombosis

As mentioned in Chapter 3, some strokes are due to blockage in the venous drainage of the brain. This type of stroke frequently causes problems in diagnosis as the symptoms are highly variable, although about 90 per cent of cases feature headache and seizures are much more common than in typical strokes. CT and magnetic resonance imaging (MRI) of the brain provides the diagnosis in this situation, although sometimes the CT appearances can be misinterpreted. The infarct will not correspond to arterial territory and is often haemorrhagic, and there are many associations with other diseases and conditions (e.g. pregnancy as described above) (see Fig. 4.3).

Patent foramen ovale (PFO)

This is a common heart anomaly affecting about a quarter of the population and is the result of incomplete fusion of parts of the heart following birth. The foramen ovale allows the fetal blood circulation to bypass the fetal lungs during life in the womb but usually completely closes in the year after birth when the baby's lungs take over oxygenation. In about a quarter of the population, the closure is incomplete but this does not cause problems for most people. Occasionally, circumstances allow blood from the right side of the heart to cross to the left side through this patent foramen ovale, and if a blood clot (or other embolus) also crosses the defect and flows to the brain, it can cause stroke. Usually, any small blood clots on the venous side of the circulation are cleared in the lung as all blood circulates from the body to the right side of the heart, to the lung, and then to the left side of the heart to be pumped around the body again, with the lung acting as a very useful sieve for debris! In some younger people, there appears to be no other risk factor for stroke apart from a PFO, and thus it is tempting to attribute the stroke to this abnormality as it is biologically plausible. It is now also possible to close this defect using a catheter technique. However, we do not yet know whether this is an effective treatment, and several large RCTs are currently underway to prove this one

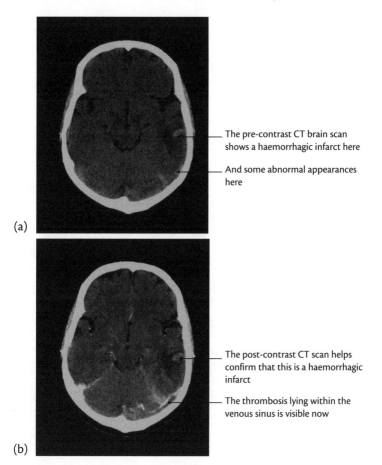

(a)

The pre-contrast CT brain scan shows a haemorrhagic infarct here

And some abnormal appearances here

(b)

The post-contrast CT scan helps confirm that this is a haemorrhagic infarct

The thrombosis lying within the venous sinus is visible now

Figure 4.3 CT scans of venous sinus thrombosis.

way or another. If it took 40 years for the first blood clot to cross the PFO, then a 40-year-old stroke patient may take a chance that the next one is due in another 40 years time! The closure of PFOs has become rather controversial, as the ability to close the defect has led to many people undergoing the procedure before we actually have reliable evidence that this is a good thing to do. To date, PFO has not satisfied the strict rules of causation (see Chapter 3) and more research is required.

5

What can be done for people who have a stroke?

 Key points

- People with suspected stroke should be assessed in hospital as soon as possible.

- The Face–Arm–Speech Test (FAST) is a helpful reminder of the common features of stroke.

- Patients with suspected stroke should have a brain scan as soon as possible after arriving at hospital.

- Treatment depends on the results on the brain scan and many other factors.

- All patients with stroke should be offered stroke unit care.

The majority of people who have a stroke are admitted to hospital. Before the modern era of brain scanning and stroke unit care, hospital admission was often reserved for people who needed care because of the disability brought on by the stroke. Nowadays, assessment in hospital concentrates on the need to make an accurate diagnosis, provide urgent treatment, identify and treat the cause of the stroke, and start the sometimes long rehabilitation road to recovery. In this chapter, I will summarize the first few hours and days of this process (see boxes).

The stroke journey

Important questions	Process
Is it a stroke?	Diagnosis
What has caused this stroke?	Investigation
What problems has the stroke caused?	Assessment
What should be done immediately?	Emergency treatment, management, and rehabilitation
What should be done later?	Rehabilitation

Recognizing stroke quickly

 Case study

A 20-year-old student collapsed in the street, very near the local emergency hospital. Her collapse was witnessed by a nearby pedestrian who immediately called an ambulance. She arrived at hospital within an hour of her collapse and, to the surprise of the emergency team, was unable to get her words out, had an obvious weakness affecting the right side of her face and her right arm and leg, and was unable to see objects in her right visual field. Subsequent tests confirmed a stroke. She had no vascular risk factors but on investigation was found to have a patent foramen ovale and an atrial septal aneurysm. In the absence of any other explanation for her stroke, this heart abnormality was the presumed to be the cause of her stroke.

 Case study

A 75-year-old lady was having breakfast with her husband when she slumped to the right. Her husband had to hold her up, but she failed to respond to his questions. Her right arm and leg were paralysed. Her husband called the ambulance and in hospital she was could only vocalize meaningless sounds, was found to have a dense right-sided weakness, and appeared not to notice objects in her right visual field. Her CT scan confirmed an ischaemic stroke, and she was found to have atrial fibrillation, the probable cause of her stroke.

 ## Case study

An 75-year-old lady complained of feeling 'funny' and then noticed that her left arm was weak and clumsy. She called her daughter, who was concerned, and she was brought to hospital. In hospital she was found to have a small cerebral infarct affecting the right side of her brain. Subsequent tests confirmed that she had a very narrowed right carotid artery. She then had a successful right carotid endarterectomy to help prevent further strokes from the tight carotid stenosis.

 ## Case study

The wife of a 45-year-old teacher heard a thump from the next room and found her husband unconscious on the floor. She called an ambulance immediately. In hospital, the CT scan showed a haemorrhagic stroke in the brainstem. Sadly, he never regained consciousness and died a few days later.

 ## Case study

A retired 70-year-old lawyer awoke with a clumsy right arm and word-finding difficulty. She had been a heavy smoker and was an enthusiastic social drinker (her words!). She made a rapid recovery and was almost back to normal by the second day. Her initial CT brain scan was normal (thus excluding haemorrhage as a cause of the stroke) but carotid duplex scanning revealed a tight left internal carotid artery stenosis. Her cholesterol was raised at 6 mmol/litre, her electrocardiogram (ECG) showed evidence of a previous heart attack, and she was found to have mild diabetes. These tests all suggested she had potent risk factors and evidence of atherosclerotic disease. She had a left carotid endarterectomy, and was discharged with medication to lower her blood pressure and cholesterol, and aspirin to thin the blood, and was strongly advised to stop smoking.

As you can see from the above stories, stroke occurs suddenly, often without warning, with features ranging from a mere clumsiness of the hand to a rapidly fatal collapse into unconsciousness. Given this bewildering range of different features, simple checklists have been developed to help guide the public into recognizing stroke and then (hopefully) getting emergency medical attention. The UK Stroke Association checklist is shown in Fig. 5.1, and similar campaigns exist elsewhere. Whilst these simple checklists do not cover all eventualities, they can help people identify stroke in a timely fashion and hopefully get expert help quickly as 'time is brain'.

Time is brain

In biochemical terms, the basic problem with the brain is that it needs a constant supply of oxygen and nutrients from the arterial blood supply, and brain cells have a limited capacity to survive if the blood supply is disrupted by a stroke. In fact, the brain starts to die within minutes of vascular occlusion or disruption. The central core of the volume of brain supplied by the artery probably dies (infarcts) within minutes; the surrounding core may survive somewhat longer (minutes to hours) depending on the alternative blood supplies (collateral vessels) to that tissue. Surprisingly for such a vital organ, the brain only has a rather rudimentary collateral blood supply in the circle of Willis, and in many people this is incomplete (Fig. 5.2). In addition, build-up of atheroma can limit this collateral blood flow even further (I have seen patients who appear to have been running successfully with only one of the four major arteries to the brain remaining open). The complex cascade of biochemical reactions that are triggered in the event of a stroke are beyond the scope of this book; suffice it to say that all attempts to intervene have so far been unsuccessful. It had been hoped that this type of treatment (neuroprotection) could buy time to allow the occluded blood vessels to be re-opened. The failure of this approach is due to two main reasons: the treatments tested do not work, or the effects of treatment have been too small to detect.

Emergency treatment of stroke

Stroke is now an eminently treatable medical emergency, and treatment in the best stroke centres offers the chance of reversing the stroke completely. Unfortunately, the pathway to successful stroke treatment is not easy, and the standard of stroke services around the world is surprisingly variable. The chief requirements are a speedy and specialist assessment to ensure that the available treatments and management strategies are correctly applied. The challenge is having such a service available 24 hours a day at all major hospitals. The most effective early medical treatment has to be given within 3 hours of stroke

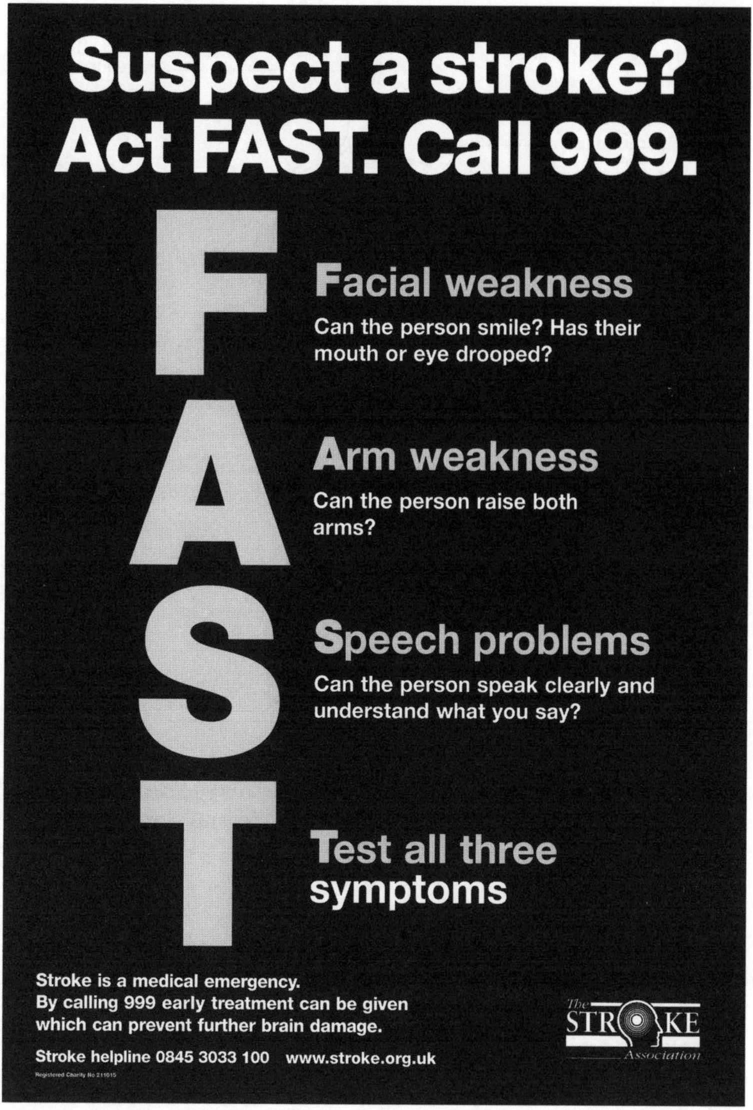

Figure 5.1 The FAST test.

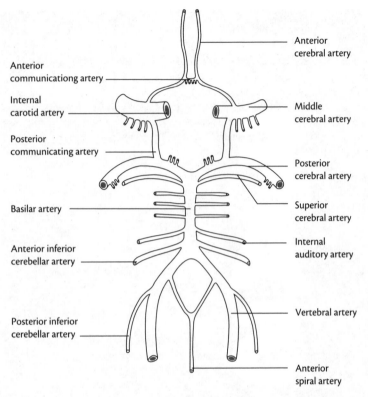

Figure 5.2 Diagram showing the main blood supply to the brain. The communicating arteries are often very small, or even absent, thus limiting potential alternative routes of blood to the brain.

onset and this sets the tone for the rest of this section – you need a first-class system to cope with the complexities.

Care at home

Some people, such as those in long-term care in a nursing home, have a stroke on the background of severely disabling disease. It may be reasonable to avoid the distress of a hospital admission for such a person. As stroke becomes more of a disease of the very frail elderly, this is likely to become a more common scenario. For others, care at home has been evaluated, but this type of service has not been shown to be better than hospital-based care in a stroke unit.

Emergency stroke pathway

Nothing can be done if medical attention is not sought, and so the immediate response to a person with suspected stroke is to call for help, and an emergency ambulance is usually the best course of action. Until fairly recently, suspected stroke did not guarantee a 'blue light' ambulance but this is now changing as ambulance service protocols start to recognize the developments in emergency stroke care. Whilst waiting for emergency transfer to hospital, people with suspected stroke should be supported by basic first aid (check the ABC of resuscitation: airway, breathing, and circulation).

Is it a stroke?

A great deal of work has been done to try and improve the recognition of stroke by the public and emergency staff. The FAST test has become widely promoted as a useful *aide-mémoire* and it has the advantage of being simple and medically correct! The FAST test is based on the fact that stroke commonly affects speech and the muscles to the face and arm, so if you suspect someone may be having a stroke ask the following questions.

Facial weakness: Can the person smile? Has their eye or mouth dropped?

Arm weakness: Can the person raise both arms?

Speech problems: Can the person speak clearly and understand what you say?

Test all symptoms (alternative versions: Time to act FAST!)

If the answer to any of the FAST questions is 'yes', a stroke is possible and an urgent ambulance should be called for. Ambulance crews should transport the patient to the nearest stroke centre with speed, ideally warning the emergency department of their imminent arrival to mobilize the stroke team. Once in the emergency room, the patient should be assessed immediately, but this is not easy as there are often competing emergencies. In addition, studies have demonstrated that about a fifth of all stroke diagnoses in a typical emergency department are incorrect, as many other conditions mimic stroke (Table 5.1). Ideally, the patient should be seen by a specialist stroke physician as soon as possible. A brief clinical assessment is all that is required to diagnose many of the mimics of stroke, but if stroke looks most likely, the next step is to get brain imaging completed.

Table 5.1 The common mimics of stroke

Epileptic seizures
Brain tumours
Migraine
Metabolic problems (e.g. low blood sugar)

Stroke mimics

 Case study

A 75-year-old man started having trouble controlling his urine whilst on holiday. A few days later his wife thought that his voice had become slurred. On their return from holiday a week later, the symptoms deteriorated and he started dribbling fluids when drinking. His GP diagnosed a minor stroke. However, over the following week, he developed some drooping of the right side of his mouth. At that point he was sent to hospital and a brain scan showed a tumour in the left part of his brain.

 Case study

A 40-year-old teacher awoke to find his speech was slurred. He was then surprised to see his appearance in the mirror – his face looked quite different from normal. His GP sent him to hospital, suspecting a stroke. His brain scan was normal and the neurologist diagnosed bilateral Bell's palsy – a curious condition where the facial nerve becomes swollen (perhaps by a viral infection or other causes) and the resulting neuropathy causes paralysis of the facial muscles. It usually only affects one side of the face, but attacks on both sides are also known. Neuropathies like Bell's palsy are potential mimics of stroke.

Ischaemic stroke or primary intracerebral haemorrhage?

Brain imaging is essential to diagnose whether a stroke is ischaemic or haemorrhagic. The basic problem is that ischaemic stroke and haemorrhagic stroke can present in exactly the same way, and only a brain scan can reliably distinguish one from the other. As further medical care treatment depends on the underlying pathology of stroke, an early brain scan is essential. There are two commonly used types of brain scan: computed tomography (CT) and magnetic resonance imaging (MRI). There is no simple answer to the question of which scan is best as each has its advantages and disadvantages (Table 5.2). Pictures of the two types of scanner and examples of the types of images obtained are shown in Figs 5.3 and 5.4. Research has shown that an early scan is cost effective, as subsequent management can be focused on the underlying pathology in a timely manner. Indeed, a delayed scan can create uncertainty, as about 1 in 100 ischaemic strokes develop massive bleeding and then look exactly like primary intracerebral haemorrhage.

What can be done immediately?

Once a diagnosis of the pathological cause of stroke is made (e.g. clinical assessment and an early brain scan) medical treatment should be considered. This differs for ischaemic stroke and primary intracerebral haemorrhage.

Ischaemic stroke

As the stroke has been caused by an arterial clot or embolus, successful treatment requires this to be removed, and removed quickly. If this can be done, some strokes can be completely reversed. This can be achieved with medical therapy such as thrombolytic treatment or mechanical therapy using an arterial clot retrieval system through a catheter inserted into the top of the leg. Thrombolysis (breaking up the clot), a routine treatment for heart attacks, has not been so widely evaluated for ischaemic stroke, although stroke trials indicate that treatment can be effective, but only if given within 3 hours of the onset of the stroke. However, there are several provisos.

◆ Few people over the age of 80 years were included in the clinical trials (and this age group now accounts for about a third of all strokes).

◆ Treatment has been surprisingly difficult to implement in many stroke centres because of the short time window (patients have to get to hospital, be assessed, complete brain scanning, and start treatment within 3 hours of stroke onset).

Table 5.2 Advantages and disadvantages of CT and MRI scanning

Advantages	Disadvantages
CT scanning	
Widely available	Can be normal in the early stages of stroke, early changes subtle
Quick (5–10 minutes)	Bone artefact limits resolution for brainstem infarcts
Haemorrhage reliably identified immediately after stroke	Haemorrhage signs disappear within days/weeks of stroke, thereafter can mimic infarct
Perfusion and angiography data can be obtained (but contrast media required)	Radiation dose with each scan
Interpretation skills widely available	Contrast media can make renal failure worse
Few contraindications	Resolution misses smaller infarcts (e.g. lacunar infarction)
Patients can be monitored easily	
MRI scanning	
Sensitive to small stroke lesions (especially brainstem)	Contraindications to scan are common (pacemakers, claustrophobia)
Advanced imaging can provide superb physiological data, e.g. identify the ischaemic penumbra	Expensive, and scanners are not so widely available
Diffusion-weighted imaging can provide early confirmation of stroke	Special sequences required for haemorrhage
No radiation	Interpretation skills less widely available
Haemorrhage can be identified months/years after stroke	Patients cannot be monitored easily
	Scan sequences and processing time longer than CT

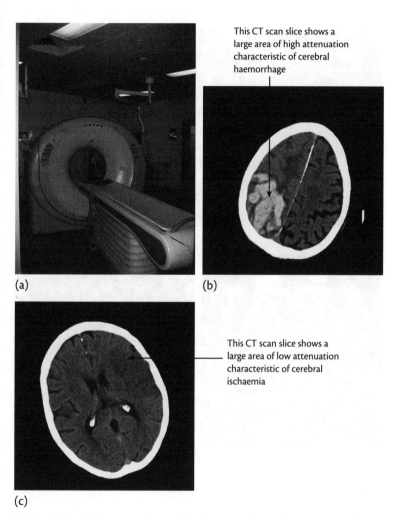

This CT scan slice shows a large area of high attenuation characteristic of cerebral haemorrhage

(a)

(b)

This CT scan slice shows a large area of low attenuation characteristic of cerebral ischaemia

(c)

Figure 5.3 (a) A CT scanner and examples of imaging showing the typical appearances of (b) haemorrhage stroke and (c) ischaemic stroke.

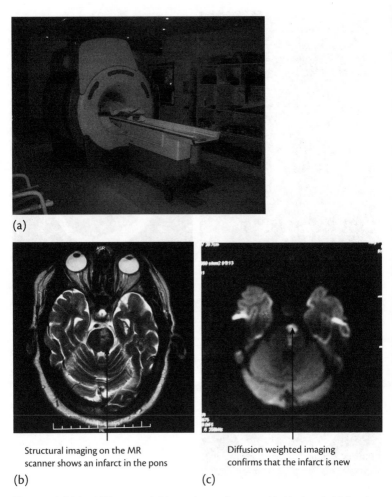

(a)

Structural imaging on the MR
scanner shows an infarct in the pons

(b)

Diffusion weighted imaging
confirms that the infarct is new

(c)

Figure 5.4 (a) An MRI scanner (with a patient well wrapped in blankets inside) and
(b, c) an example of imaging showing a small cerebral infarct in the pons of the brain.

- The treatment has an unusually high risk of complications (bleeding in the brain).

- Audits have shown that treatment in routine clinical practice may not always be as successful as in the randomized controlled trials (RCTs).

As a result, this treatment is still the subject of much research to try and improve safety, to improve stroke thrombolysis provision, to test thrombolysis treatment in older people and those presenting later than 3 hours, and to identify novel approaches (e.g. intravenous and then intra-arterial therapy).

Unfortunately, even the best stroke centres in the world struggle to treat 10–20 per cent of patients with thrombolysis, and this figure is very much lower in most centres and countries.

Intra-arterial and interventional treatment

In intra-arterial treatment a specialist neuroradiologist inserts a catheter into the blood vessel system at the groin (a bit like a coronary angiogram) and threads a fine catheter into the blocked artery in the brain. Dye is then injected to confirm the blockage followed by a thrombolytic (clot-dissolving) drug to try and unblock the artery. This is impressive when the artery can be seen to re-open with successful therapy. However, this has only been feasible for a tiny proportion of patients as this degree of expertise is usually only available in very large or specialized urban hospitals. Mechanical clot removal is now possible with a variety of ingenious catheter devices inserted in the same way, but the bleeding complications appear to be similar to those associated with thrombolysis treatment, presumably because of mechanical trauma to the cerebral vessels and the fact that the brain bleeds easily. Because of current regulations, there has not been a strict requirement for reliable RCTs for these clot removal catheters and thus it is uncertain whether these devices offer any benefit over medical treatment such as thrombolysis. This type of high-tech treatment will only be available for the few for the foreseeable years.

Thrombolysis and mechanical clot retrieval both require a sophisticated and organized emergency stroke service which is often not available. In the absence of these treatments, the mainstay of immediate treatment is aspirin. Aspirin has been extensively tested in RCTs worldwide, with over 40 000 patients included in the major studies. These trials have clearly shown that aspirin, at a starting dose of 160–300 milligrams a day, has important, albeit modest, benefits. For about every 100 patients treated, there is one extra independent survivor in the first 2 weeks of treatment. Put another way, aspirin given for 2 weeks in the acute phase of ischaemic stroke has the same benefits as the next 50 weeks of secondary prevention (see Chapter 8).

In public health terms the current use of aspirin has far greater benefit than more effective treatments such as thrombolysis. This is because aspirin, with only a modest yet definite benefit, can be given to virtually everybody with ischaemic stroke. Good old aspirin will have a much greater public health impact than thrombolysis for many years to come unless stroke thrombolysis rates can reach about 10–20 per cent of all ischaemic strokes.

No other medical treatments have been shown to have definite benefits for ischaemic stroke – and many have been evaluated. For further details on these, readers are referred to the Cochrane Library (see box) which has an excellent stroke section. Blood-thinning treatment with immediate anticoagulation has been extensively used in the past, and on the face of it appears to be a logical treatment. If the stroke is due to a blood clot, an anticoagulant would seem to be a sensible treatment. However, despite a large number of trials, testing many different anticoagulation regimens, a similar pattern has emerged. Immediate anticoagulation with drugs such as heparin decreases the early risk of having another ischaemic stroke, but this benefit is balanced by a small but definite increase in having an early haemorrhagic stroke. The two cancel each other out with no net benefit. Anticoagulation was widely used before these data became available and is still popular with some neurologists! However, most stroke physicians only use immediate anticoagulation cautiously for selected patients, and the risks of haemorrhagic transformation of the infarct should be kept in mind.

The Cochrane Library

The Cochrane Library is an electronic archive of systematic reviews of RCTs of thousands of different interventions. It addresses criticism of the medical profession by Archie Cochrane (1909–1988) who wrote in 1979: 'It is surely a great criticism of our profession that we have not organized a critical summary, by specialty or subspecialty, adapted periodically, of all relevant randomized controlled trials'.

A systematic review statistically summarizes the results of different RCTs of similar interventions to provide a more reliable estimate of the balance of risks and benefits of treatments. It was found that, for many treatments, individual trials were not large enough to provide clear answers, but a systematic review of all the trials often identified an important benefit (or risk).

Some researchers (myself included) have compared the importance of the Cochrane Library with the Human Genome Project, such is its value. In fact, the data within the Cochrane Library have probably been responsible for improving the health care of some hundreds of millions of patients to date.

The future is exciting for stroke treatment as new technologies are providing a whole new armamentarium of possibilities ranging from nanomolecules to ultrasound dissolution of blood clots. One disappointing aspect of stroke medicine is the failure of the researchers to design really large RCTs to reliably rule in, or rule out, promising treatments for stroke. The cardiologists learnt this message two decades ago, but since the two 'mega-trials' of aspirin for acute ischaemic stroke completed in the mid 1990s, no further stroke 'mega-trials' have been planned.

Surgical treatment for ischaemic stroke

The brain is effectively in a closed box (the skull) and any condition that causes it to swell carries extreme risks for the patient as the swelling can rapidly lead to brain death. Very large ischaemic strokes can lead to fatal brain swelling by this mechanism. Typically, these types of stroke are due to occlusion of the middle cerebral artery which can lead to swelling affecting a third of the brain. Older people, by virtue of their age-related brain atrophy, have more potential space to accommodate this brain swelling, but in younger people this type of stroke can rapidly be fatal. In fact the medical term: 'malignant middle cerebral artery infarction' reflects the seriousness of the condition. In an effort to treat this severe complication, neurosurgeons have been performing decompressive surgery, literally removing a large piece of the skull to allow the brain to swell outwards and not cause herniation and brainstem death. Whilst many commentators have considered this treatment rather crude, with a potential to save life but leave the survivors with severe disability, recent research has suggested that somewhat against expectation, this sort of heroic surgery can not only save lives but also improve the chances of surviving with less severe disability. An overview of the early results from three trials (called DECIMAL, DESTINY, and HAMLET) indicated that surgery reduced deaths by 50 per cent and also increased survival with moderate to mild disability. As a result of these important RCTs, neurosurgeons now have the necessary information about the potential risks and benefits of this procedure when discussing this operation with patients, relatives, and their carers. This will remain a rare intervention, but the size of the benefit for patients under 60 years of age suggests that older people may also derive some benefit. This will no doubt be the focus of further research.

Case study

A 40-year-old farm worker was admitted to hospital with a sudden weakness of his left face, arm, and leg. On examination he had no power at all on his left-hand side (a left dense hemiparesis), he could not see to the left (left homonymous hemianopia), and he was ignoring objects on the left (left-sided inattention). He was apathetic and became increasingly drowsy over the following 24 hours. His initial CT scan showed a right middle cerebral artery infarct, and a repeat CT at 24 hours showed swelling of the entire right hemisphere of the brain. The neurosurgeons were consulted and agreed that decompressive surgery may save his life. At surgery his brain was indeed very swollen and dramatically filled the space where his skull had been removed. After a period of intensive care, he was transferred to rehabilitation and after 6 weeks he had started to walk. He turned out to be an illegal immigrant, and when he was deported to his home country he carried the piece of skull that was removed in his hand-luggage with a note to customs explaining the importance of his keeping this piece of bone, in case it was to be replaced in future years!

Primary intracerebral haemorrhage (PICH)

The treatment of PICH stroke (or haemorrhagic stroke) has changed rapidly in recent years. Traditionally, the mainstay of treatment was supportive care and surgical removal of the blood for selected patients. Investigations were then performed to exclude an underlying cause of the bleed such as a cerebral aneurysm. The role of surgery was examined in a large pragmatic RCT involving over 1000 patients and early surgical evacuation of the haematoma was not found to be beneficial compared with best medical care. This does not mean that there is no role for surgery as one of the exclusion criteria was 'definite need for surgery', but the trial strongly suggested that surgery was not a beneficial option for a large proportion of patients with haemorrhagic stroke. Selected use of neurosurgery still has a place and will depend on individual factors (see box).

Possible indications for surgical evacuation of haematoma for patients with primary intracerebral haemorrhage

◆ Cerebellar haemorrhage causing acute hydrocephalus

◆ Rapidly deteriorating condition in young patient

◆ Peripheral haematoma

Haemorrhagic stroke due to anticoagulation

Nowadays, there is much more proactive treatment of PICH stroke in cases due to over-anticoagulation with treatment such as warfarin. This has been helped by new blood-clotting factor medication such as recombinant activated Factor VII (aFVII), which can be injected together with vitamin K. This treatment works by restoring the ability of the blood to clot normally. Rapid reversal of any clotting disorder is thought to be beneficial in the emergency situation of a PICH stroke as we know that the haematoma causing the stroke grows rapidly in the first few hours after stroke onset, and any reduction in the eventual size of the haematoma will reduce the severe consequences of this type of stroke. aFVII acts very quickly, and vitamin K reverses the effects of blood-thinning treatment with warfarin but has an effect that is much slower (many hours to days). However, this new method of reversing the blood-clotting disorder has not been subject to the rigours of an RCT comparing treatment with the older methods of providing the missing clotting by a transfusion of fresh frozen plasma and vitamin K injections.

aFVII is also a promising treatment for the medical treatment of PICH. In two large international RCTs, treatment with aFVII limited the expansion of the haematoma. In the first trial, treatment was associated with a better clinical outcome. In the second trial, called the FAST trial, there was no clinical benefit with treatment. It is likely that aFVII does work, but perhaps more modestly than the researchers estimated. A larger trial will be required to confirm these promising initial results.

Admission to the stroke unit

Once urgent medical and surgical treatment has been considered (see above), admission to a stroke unit has been shown to be better than care in a general ward. Despite the publication of numerous RCTs of stroke unit care, the medical profession was largely ignorant of these benefits until a systematic review of all the trials was published. This is a nice example of the power of this type of review (see page 60). Individually, few of the stroke unit trials were statistically significant in their own right, but when they were reviewed as a whole, the substantial benefits of stroke unit care became apparent. For every 100 patients admitted to a comprehensive or rehabilitation stroke unit, there are six more independent survivors, seven fewer people in institutional care, and five fewer deaths. There are few medical treatments that can match the magnitude of this benefit. Furthermore, these benefits are not at the cost of extra days in hospital. How do stroke units work? Well, the answer is probably because of the numerous simple interventions done well by a specialized and educated multidisciplinary team. Typically, these may include the following:

◆ correct positioning of paralysed limbs

◆ early assessment by all members of a specialized stroke team including nurses, physiotherapists, occupational therapists, social workers, medical staff, and speech therapists, often augmented by dieticians, pharmacists, and psychologists

◆ good hydration with an intravenous drip (usually containing normal saline)

◆ scrupulous bowel and bladder care and avoidance of urinary catheterization wherever possible

◆ early mobilization

◆ strategies to prevent deep vein thrombosis (DVT)

◆ involvement of family members and other carers in the recovery process

◆ regular team meetings

◆ provision of individualized information and advice.

Crucial early assessments by the team will include swallow assessments to ensure that patients at risk of aspirating food or fluid are prescribed a modified diet or kept nil by mouth. Medical assessment will include further tests to try and answer the question: Why has this person had a stroke? These early investigations will identify treatable risk, may identify the cause of stroke, and enable early use of secondary preventative measures.

Why has this person had a stroke?

The exact profile of tests usually depends on the pathology of stroke (infarct of haemorrhage) and the condition of the patient.

In people with primary intracerebral haemorrhage, further tests will often involve:

◆ selected further brain imaging (e.g. cerebral angiography) to identify any underlying lesion such as cerebral aneurysm or arteriovenous malformation

◆ blood clotting screen to detect delayed clotting tendency due to disease (e.g. liver failure) or medication (e.g. warfarin).

In people with cerebral ischaemia, investigations are focused on what has caused the arterial occlusion. This will involve some or all of the following:

◆ electrocardiogram (ECG) to detect atrial fibrillation, left ventricular hypertrophy, and recent myocardial infarction

◆ 24-hour ECG monitoring to detect paroxysmal atrial fibrillation

◆ chest X-ray to determine heart size and potential general medical problems

◆ fasting blood glucose to detect diabetes mellitus

◆ blood cholesterol

◆ echocardiography to detect intracardiac thrombosis, heart lesions, or aortic arch disease, all of which will cause cardio-embolic stroke

◆ carotid duplex scanning to detect carotid stenosis

◆ thrombophilia screen to detect blood clotting tendency in younger people

◆ syphilis serology (an unusual cause of stroke)

◆ blood cultures to detect bacterial endocarditis (unusual cause of stroke).

After stroke has been confirmed, the initial assessments have been completed, and medical investigations ordered, the best place for the patient is a stroke unit. What happens next depends on many factors, but perhaps the most important is what effect the stroke has had on the patient. A review of some of the different types of stroke, and what can happen next is the focus of the next chapter.

Further reading

Anonymous (1997) Collaborative systematic review of the randomised trials of organised inpatient (stroke unit) care after stroke. Stroke Unit Trialists' Collaboration. *British Medical Journal*, **314**, 1151.

Cochrane Library. Summaries of the aspirin, thrombolysis, stroke unit and anticoagulation trials are available online at: http://www3.interscience.wiley.com/cgi-bin/mrwhome/106568753/HOME?CRETRY=1&SRETRY=0 (the library is available free to many nationalities including the UK and Australia).

Mayer SA, Brun NC, Begtrup K, *et al.* (2005) Recombinant activated Factor VII for acute intracerebral hemorrhage. *New England Journal of Medicine*, **35**, 777–85.

Mendelow AD, Gregson BA, Fernandes HM, *et al.* (2005) Early surgery versus initial conservative treatment in patients with spontaneous supratentorial intracerebral haematomas in the International Surgical Trial in Intracerebral Haemorrhage (STICH): a randomised trial. *Lancet*, **365**, 387–97.

Vahedi K, Hofmeijer J, Juettler E, *et al.* (2007) Early decompressive surgery in malignant infarction of the middle cerebral artery: a pooled analysis of three randomised controlled trials. *Lancet Neurology*, **3**, 215–22.

6

Rehabilitation after stroke

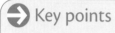 Key points

♦ Every person's stroke is unique; therefore rehabilitation must be an individualized process.

♦ Organized stroke unit care achieves the best outcome.

During the initial stages of stroke most people are in a state of shock and bewilderment. For those admitted to hospital, the first few days are a blur of tests and assessments by numerous health professionals (see previous chapter for an outline of the initial priorities). There will come a time when the person with a stroke will take stock and consider their position. It is hard to give a general example as stroke can cause so many different situations. The large range in stroke severity is important to understand. In a typical stroke service, about 10–20 per cent of those admitted will have such severe strokes that they will die as a result. About half of the survivors will have mild symptoms that will enable a very quick discharge, usually within a few days or a week, but the remainder of the early survivors will need rehabilitation because of the severity of their problems. To understand what these problems are, it is worth discussing some basic neuro-anatomy and getting a feel for the workings of the brain.

The World Health Organization has developed a model of illness on which to base discussions of stroke rehabilitation (Fig. 6.1). In the last chapter we talked about the pathology – the stroke. We now need to consider what effects the stroke has on the body – this is called impairment.

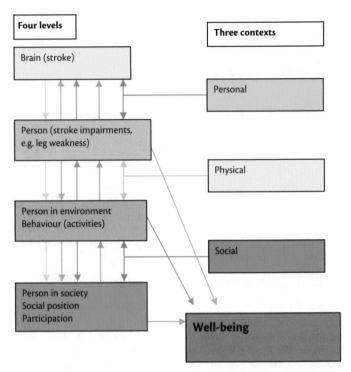

Figure 6.1 World Health Organization International Classification of Function: a useful model of stroke rehabilitation. (Adapted with permission from Derick Wade).

Stroke impairment

To start with, we need to see what the brain looks like (Figs 6.2 and 6.3). In structural terms, I like to describe the brain in terms of the 'computer processor' and the 'wiring'. The 'computer processor' is the complex interaction of brain cells, called neurons, which look grey if you cut a real brain, hence their colloquial term 'grey matter'. This neural grey matter is concentrated in the outermost layer of the cerebral hemispheres of the brain. The 'wiring' is the neuronal connections which connect different parts of the brain; a large bundle connects the right brain to the left brain, and another large bundle carries the messages down to the spinal cord and receives messages from the body up the spinal cord. In addition, specific areas of the brain control different functions essential for life. The centres that control breathing, for example, are in the base of the brain – the brainstem. If that centre is damaged by a stroke,

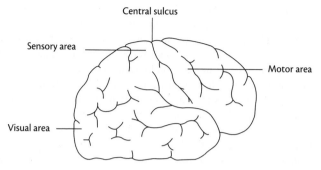

Figure 6.2 Lateral view of the brain showing the motor, visual, and sensory areas.

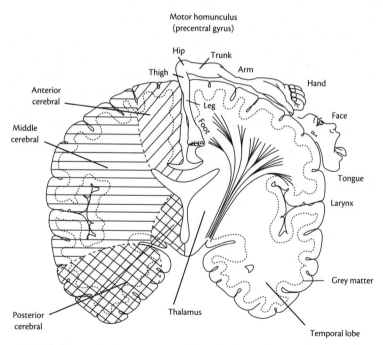

Figure 6.3 Diagram of the motor cortex of the brain showing the position of the grey matter responsible for different areas of the body – the homunculus.

then the stroke will be rapidly fatal. The reticular formation, an interconnecting system of fibres in the brainstem and the mid-brain, controls consciousness; if that is affected, the stroke can cause coma. The right hemispheres generally control the left body functions (and vice versa). Language function – our ability to communicate by voice and writing – is usually localized in the dominant hemisphere, which in most people is the left hemisphere. The vast majority of right-handed people, and about half of left-handed people are left-brain dominant. More detailed mapping of cerebral function has been performed for many years, and is constantly being refined using functional magnetic resonance imaging. The localization of brain function is best understood by looking at a cartoon-like representation of the brain, called the homunculus, which shows which bit of the brain controls which part of the body (Fig. 6.3). Damage to the motor cortex by stroke is responsible for the severe physical problems that arise. Muscles are weakened, there is a lack of control, tone is increased and may become particularly troublesome for some patients, and arm and leg reflexes become brisk.

If we now put this very quick and grossly simplified lesson in neuro-anatomy together with our knowledge of the blood supply to the brain, we can start to understand the stereotyped patterns of problems arising from stroke. It is easier to start understanding these concepts by considering the likely stroke problems when particular blood vessels become blocked, i.e. ischaemic stroke. PICH stroke, by virtue of the spread of blood in the haematoma, does not necessarily follow the same patterns of stroke deficit, and this can often be a clue that you are dealing with a bleed rather than an ischaemic stroke. In the 1980s a group of researchers in Oxford summarized the main patterns of stroke problems (deficits) arising from ischaemic stroke, and this classification is in widespread use in hospitals in the UK and beyond. This Oxfordshire Community Stroke Project (OCSP) classification helps us understand the main impairments associated with different sorts of strokes and divides ischaemic stroke into four main groups:

- total anterior circulation infarct (TACI)

- partial anterior circulation infarct (PACI)

- lacunar infarct (LACI)

- posterior circulation infarct (POCI).

Total anterior circulation infarct (TACI)

A TACI stroke is a large stroke due to occlusion of a large blood vessel of the brain, usually the main stem of the middle cerebral artery, but a similar deficit can occur when the blockage occurs in the internal carotid artery (Chapter 4, Fig. 4.1). A stroke causing such an occlusion leads to a large volume of brain becoming ischaemic, and in time this affected area will die. Unfortunately, the blood supply to this part of the brain is nearly all through this one main blood vessel. There may be small interconnections with other blood vessels over the surface of the brain and at the periphery of the middle cerebral artery territory, but these 'collateral' blood vessels are rarely adequate to ensure survival of this part of the brain. Over the minutes and hours following a middle cerebral artery occlusion, the brain dies from the central core outwards, leaving a very large deficit if untreated.

The consequences of such a stroke are major. A TACI stroke will include the cortical areas, the 'computer chip' parts of the brain controlling motor power, and thus will lead to paralysis of the face, arm, and leg of the opposite side of the body, termed a hemiparesis or hemiplegia. In addition, the 'computer chip' of the parts of the brain controlling sensation may be affected, leading to lack of sensation on the opposite side of the body. The nerve fibres leading from the optic nerve of the eye to the 'computer chip' for vision travel though the deep areas of the middle cerebral artery territory, and thus the field of vision on the opposite side of the body is lost. This is termed a homonymous hemianopia – homonymous because the pattern of deficit is the same for each eye, and hemianopia because the deficit is half the visual field. The major problem resulting from this type of stroke depends on the brain hemisphere affected and the 'handedness' of the person. For example, if the person is right-handed and left-brain dominant, and the stroke has affected the left brain, a TACI stroke causes a problem of language production and understanding called **aphasia** (see box). The control of language can be damaged in a stroke so that the production of correct words and language is impaired; this is called **expressive aphasia**. The problem of understanding language is called **receptive aphasia**. A good analogy of receptive aphasia is when we listen to an unfamiliar language (e.g. Mandarin Chinese); we know people are talking to each other but we cannot understand a single word. In contrast, people with expressive aphasia know what they want to say but simply cannot get the correct words out. We will discuss the management of aphasia later in the chapter.

Aphasia and dysphasia

It used to be taught that a complete loss of language is called 'aphasia', and a partial loss is called 'dysphasia', but much to the dismay of classical scholars both types of deficit are now referred to as 'aphasia'.

Language is a complex brain function, and thus is localized to the grey matter or 'computer chip' of the brain. Language requires that: a vocabulary is learnt, stored in the brain, and associated with particular sounds; rules determine how words are combined (grammar); the meaning of words is known (semantics); words express appropriate feelings (pragmatics); words are said with appropriate intonation and emphasis (prosody); appropriate computer programs of production are known for sound (requiring speech apparatus including the mouth, tongue, pharynx, and breathing) and writing (requiring appropriate dexterity of the arm, hand, and fingers with intact vision). This requires a large amount of brain power and therefore large regions of the brain.

If the TACI stroke occurs in the non-dominant brain hemisphere, for example in the right hemisphere of a right-handed person, major language skills are preserved but the person often has major problems in perceiving the left side of their personal space and world, termed visuospatial disorders. A mild version of this can present as the patient ignoring obvious visual or touch stimuli on the affected side of the body, but a severe manifestation of this can be a total unawareness of the major problems of a stroke, which is called anosognosia.

 Patient's perspective

An elderly lady was admitted to the emergency room because her home help had found her collapsed on the bedroom floor and 'confused'. When she was assessed by the stroke unit doctor, she had a very obvious left-sided weakness affecting her face, arm and leg, to the extent that she had no movement at all on that side. She was unable to see the doctors when they examined her on her left side. When asked what problems had led her to be admitted to hospital, she was bemused and stated that it was absolutely ridiculous that she had been dragged to hospital, as she felt fine and people were making a fuss about nothing. When the doctor pointed out that the left side of her body was completely paralysed, she still denied there was a problem! These types of stroke can be particularly hazardous for people as they do not obtain urgent medical attention (and are often not in any physical state to do so), and when they do get to hospital they need careful management as they are at high risk of falling out of bed and chairs.

Other common additional neurological problems from this type of stroke include brain swelling (see Chapter 5), slurred speech, difficulty in swallowing, and incontinence of urine and faeces.

Therefore TACI strokes are characterized by major impairments of weakness (hemiparesis), language or visuospatial problems, and loss of half the visual field. Not surprisingly, this represents the worst type of ischaemic stroke and carries a poor prognosis. About a fifth of people will die from this type of stroke within the first month, and at 6 months the majority (90 per cent) of people with a TACI stroke will have died or remain disabled.

Partial anterior circulation infarcts

As the name implies, this type of stroke include many but not all of the TACI problems, representing a milder version of a TACI by virtue of the arterial occlusion being further downstream and thus affecting a smaller volume of brain. A close study of Fig. 6.3 will reveal that there numerous different symptoms can result from a smaller type of stroke in the anterior circulation. Problems may be as mild as some loss of strength in one hand, or merely word-finding difficulty (mild expressive aphasia), but can include more major combinations of symptoms such as complete hemiparesis and aphasia, or a quarter loss of visual field, arm weakness, and slurred speech. PACI strokes will usually involve the 'computer chip' grey matter of the brain, and so higher cerebral functions such as language, visuospatial problems, weakness, and loss of sensation can be expected.

Important impairments usually arising from PACI or TACI strokes

Different types of aphasia

Wernicke's aphasia

This is often called receptive aphasia as understanding of language is impaired. It is also called a 'fluent aphasia' because speech occurs without hesitation but words are often used incorrectly, and there is an emptiness of speech, often gibberish, and occurrence of words that do not exist (neologisms). The stroke lesion causing Wernicke's aphasia is usually in the dominant (left-sided in most people) temporal lobe.

Broca's aphasia

This is also commonly called expressive aphasia as the production of speech is the main abnormality. It is also called a 'non-fluent aphasia' because the production of speech is very abnormal with hesitation, limited vocabulary, short sentences, poor grammar, and frequent use of the wrong words (semantic errors). The stroke lesion causing Broca's aphasia is usually in the dominant frontal lobe.

Global aphasia

This is a combination of Broca's and Wernicke's aphasias and is a very severe language impairment caused by a major dominant hemisphere stroke.

Nominal aphasia

A person with nominal aphasia can understand speech and speak reasonably well but has great difficulty in naming objects or people.

Conduction aphasia

Naming and repetition of speech is impaired. This condition is caused by a stroke lesion in a connecting nerve fibre bundle such as the arcuate fasciculus.

Apraxias

We rely on a 'computer program' in the brain to coordinate patterns of movement of muscles for everyday movements such as walking, combing our hair, or washing our hands. Sometimes individual muscles are able to move but the stroke has damaged the complex brain memory of these common movements. This will cause clumsiness when the person attempts the task and can be extremely disabling. It is obviously made much worse if it is combined with a muscle weakness due to a stroke hemiparesis. Apraxias can also make aphasias much more disabling if the person has trouble miming their requirements when rendered speechless by a stroke.

Alexia

This is a disorder of reading which can occur with a stroke.

Agraphia

This is a disorder of writing.

Lacunar infarction

Lacunar infarcts are so-called because many years after the stroke all that's left is a small hole in the brain. Lacunar infarction differ from other strokes in several important ways. First, the stroke affects the white matter of the brain, 'the wiring' and thus has no affect on mental ability. This is not to say that these strokes are trivial, unfortunately they are not, as damage to the main conduction fibres controlling, say, motor signals to the face, arm and leg, can lead to a severe paralysis. Secondly, these strokes are due to blockage of blood vessels called end-arteries, in effect a blood vessel cul de sac, which, once blocked, result in a small spherical or ovoid infarct. The third way lacunar strokes differ from other types of stroke is that the pathology of the blockage is still subject to much debate. It is possible that mechanisms other than atheroma cause the lacunar infarct, and this is still the subject of ongoing medical research. As lacunar strokes are small (but not in their effects) and affect only white matter, people with this type of stroke are spared some of the life-threatening complications of other types of stroke. For example, lacunar stroke does not cause dangerous brain oedema, and thus there is a much lower chance of dying from such a stroke. When early death occurs after a lacunar stroke, this is often due to other conditions which accompany stroke, such as a heart attack, or may be a result of the disability which follows a lacunar stroke. Finally, lacunar stroke has attracted great interest as characteristic syndromes arise from the stroke.

Lacunar syndromes

As lacunar stroke is caused by small deep lesions in the white matter of the brain, the syndromes arise as a result of the manner in which these nerve fibres are bundled together. For example, the descending nerve fibres carrying information from the motor cortex to the spinal cord come together in an area called the internal capsule. In the internal capsule, the fibres carrying motor information to the muscles of one side of the face are next to the fibres that carry motor information to the arm, which are next to the fibres that carry information to the leg. These fibres are tightly packed together, and thus neurologists noted that small deep lacunar lesions usually caused a stroke affecting all three tracts, thus causing hemiparesis (weakness of the face, arm, and leg). Smaller lacunar infarcts could perhaps cause a weak face and arm, or a weak arm and leg, but in this example they would never cause a weak face and leg, sparing the arm, as the arm fibres are between the face and the leg fibres. This type of observation led to the description of the classical lacunar syndromes (see box). With the advent of modern brain imaging, these syndromes are good at predicting the likelihood of a small deep infarct. Some cortical strokes (PACIs) can be mistaken clinically for lacunar syndromes; thus brain imaging will refine the clinical estimate of the localization of the stroke.

Classical lacunar syndromes

◆ Pure motor stroke (weakness of face, arm, and leg)

◆ Pure sensory stroke (loss of sensation in face, arm, and leg)

◆ Sensorimotor stroke (a combination of the above two syndromes)

◆ Ataxic hemisparesis (mild hemiparesis and major unsteadiness)

◆ Dysarthria clumsy hand

Posterior circulation infarct (POCI)

The posterior circulation is supplied by the pair of vertebral arteries which combine to form the basilar artery, the branches of which define 'posterior circulation'. Brain regions supplied by the posterior circulation include the occipital lobes (which process data from the eyes via the optic radiation nerve tracts), the cerebellum (important for smooth organized movement), and the brainstem. The brainstem consists of all the nerve fibres (the 'wiring') from the spinal cord carrying, for example, sensory data from the body, the motor tracts from the brain to the muscles, and many different collections of nerve centres with vital functions such as control of breathing (the respiratory centre) and control of balance and equilibrium (the vestibular nuclei). In addition, there is a special network of neurons, the reticular activating system, that are vital for maintaining consciousness. As will be appreciated from the above, strokes in this region of the brain can cause a myriad of different syndromes. These syndromes were often named after the neurologist who first described them and are numerous! A few examples are shown in the box. With the advent of sensitive brain scans such as MRI, it has been found that these syndromes are virtually never 'pure' and there can be remarkable variability in symptoms between people with similar lesions on the scan.

Some posterior circulation infarct syndromes named after the neurologist who first described them

Lateral medullary syndrome of Wallenburg

Ipsilateral Horner's syndrome (descending sympathetic nerve fibres)

Contralateral limb loss of pain and temperature (ascending spinothalamic tract)

Ipsilateral facial palsy (descending trigeminal tract)

Vertigo, nausea, vomiting, and nystagmus (vertibular nuclei)

Ipsilateral ataxia of the limbs (inferior cerebellar peduncle)

Ipsilateral paralysis of the palate, larynx, and pharynx causing dysphonia, dysarthria, and dysphagia (nucleus ambiguus)

Benedikt's syndrome

Cerebellar ataxia

Third cranial nerve palsy

Weber's syndrome

Third nerve palsy

Hemiplegia of the opposite side

Strokes affecting the cerebellum classically cause an unsteadiness called ataxia, familiar to everyone who has seen a drunk walk (acute alcohol intoxication causes cerebellar dysfunction).

A major stroke affecting the brainstem can rapidly lead to death if the vital centres are affected (e.g. an arterial occlusion of the basilar artery), and less severe strokes can cause a decreased level of consciousness. The mechanism of death from large TACI strokes (malignant middle cerebral artery syndrome) is due to the compression of the brainstem when the brain hemisphere herniates.

Symptoms due to PICH

Some PICH strokes present in identical manner to the TACI/PACI/LACI/ POCI subtypes described above if the bleed is in a similar part of the brain. For example, a small deep bleed in the internal capsule will cause a lacunar syndrome of pure motor stroke, but the brain imaging will identify that this has been due to a small bleed rather than an infarct. One additional complication of lacunar disease is that the small-vessel pathology that causes occlusion can just as easily lead to vessel rupture, and thus infarct and haemorrhage may have the same underlying pathology (which contrasts with haemorrhages elsewhere).

Other PICH strokes present in ways that differ from the subtypes of cerebral infarction described above in that the presentation is often more apoplectic (e.g. a catastrophic collapse and quick decline in consciousness) and the patient is often drowsier, especially if the blood has escaped into the surroundings of the brain (subarachnoid spread) or if the haematoma is rapidly expanding, causing compression of vital structures in the brainstem. The spread of blood across usual vascular territory can give rise to combinations of symptoms that are difficult to place in the OCSP classification system.

However, despite these general rules, the underlying pathology of stroke (infarct versus haemorrhage) cannot be identified unless an early brain scan is done.

Other comments on the impairments arising from stroke

A few key concepts are worth considering. Strokes cause the brain to stop working and thus most of the features of stroke consist of negative symptoms, for example weakness, loss of vision, loss of balance, or loss of feeling. Positive symptoms, such as flashing lights and pins and needles, can often point to other causes of neurological disease (e.g. migraine or nerve entrapment, respectively). A trap for the unwary is the common use of language by the patient that does not conform to the medical definition of the same term. For example, people will often say that their arm became numb, but they are referring to weakness. Dizziness, vertigo, giddiness, lightheadedness, and 'coming over queer' may all refer to the hallucination of movement called vertigo, but careful dissection of common language is required!

Another trap for the unwary is lack of recognition of the diversity of the vascular supply to the brain. There is enormous anatomical variation between individuals, and also over time in individuals. Parts of the brain that are supplied by the posterior circulation in one person are supplied by the anterior circulation in others. In some people, the accumulating atheroma in the blood supply to the brain can lead to them managing on three, two, or even one of the usual four main blood supplies to the brain (the two vertebral arteries and the two internal carotid arteries). For such individuals, occlusion of the remaining single arterial supply to the brain will result in rapid death. This is important because it means that the 'rules' for stroke symptoms given above will have variability amongst individuals, further complicating any description of a typical stroke. We are all individuals and every stroke will be different, and if we then add the differing personal, social, and physical contexts of stroke, together with the differing pathology, person, environment, and position in society, it is obvious that rehabilitation must be conducted on a person by person basis (see Fig. 6.1).

Rehabilitation after stroke

We now need to consider where we are in the stroke journey. We have confirmed that the nature of the problem is a stroke, we have established the pathology, investigations are underway, and emergency treatment has been given. Without doubt the best place to be for most people is in a specialized stroke unit. This would appear to be such an obvious statement, that some people wonder why it is such an issue. Surely, we would all want the best specialized care if struck down by a major illness? The fact is that stroke units are, medically speaking, a new phenomenon and have yet to be widely implemented in many countries. This is despite the fact that for every 1000 people treated in a stroke unit, there are an extra 56 independent survivors which, medically speaking, is an impressive result. In Chapter 5 we discussed some of the reasons why stroke units are effective, but the most obvious reason is that a large number of different things must be done in a short period of time to help rescue the brain and get the patient on the road to recovery. My own personal view, increasingly supported by research, is that rehabilitation should start immediately, and certainly within the first few days of admission. However, there is still debate about this, and I was bemused to read of an eminent stroke neurologist who was recommending a few days of bed rest as recently as 2006! As in all things medical, this issue is being resolved by further research evaluating early and intense rehabilitation compared with the more leisurely pace seen in many units. The sad fact is that millions of people around the world do not have any rehabilitation after stroke, and, for many patients, rehabilitation is something to wait for in the acute hospital. The evidence strongly suggests that care in a comprehensive stroke unit, which offers acute assessment together with rehabilitation, achieves the best results.

Successful stroke rehabilitation

To achieve good rehabilitation results, a large team of healthcare professionals need to work with the patient, with the patient's family and carers, and with each other. The care needs to be co-ordinated, and patient-guided goals need to be determined and monitored and adapted in a flexible model of care. The basic team members are:

- medical staff

- nursing staff

- physiotherapists

- speech pathologists

- occupational therapists

- social workers.

Depending on resources, this team should also include dieticians, pharmacists, and clinical psychologists.

There is large variation in actual team membership between countries. For example, in some teams the physiotherapists perform many of the duties of an occupational therapist. Where speech therapists are in short supply, nursing staff will undertake swallow assessments to identify if the patient is at risk of aspiration pneumonia because of a disordered swallow mechanism. Differing social security systems will increase or decrease the importance of social workers. In the UK they have a key role in organizing post-discharge care and support.

Each team member will assess the patient with stroke, and each will have their own roles in the immediate care of the patient. For example, the nursing staff will ensure that the patient is positioned correctly (often guided by the physiotherapist) and in particular will attend to continence issues. This is in addition to providing 24-hour care. The physiotherapists will determine what the patient is capable of doing, and organize therapy (training) to improve activities. The occupational therapists will determine the patient's abilities to perform basic activities of life such as washing, dressing, and feeding. Speech therapists (often called speech pathologists) have established a role for assessing swallow function as well as speech. Dieticians have a crucial role to play if the patient needs to be tube fed for a period. A good team will blur their professional roles to allow more seamless care, and careful coordination is required. Many of the best teams will meet daily, albeit briefly, with more detailed discussion saved for formal multidisciplinary meetings or individual meetings for particular patients.

An important role of the team is to provide holistic care, which realistically develops important goals for the patient and their family, whilst screening for stroke complications and trouble-shooting as problems present. Given the increasing age of patients with stroke, it is very common for people to have multiple medical problems. Patients often have pre-existing disability from non-stroke conditions, and the co-ordination of medical care is as important as the physical rehabilitation.

How does rehabilitation work?

It used to be believed that rehabilitation merely facilitated the natural improvement of stroke with time. What was damaged was irretrievably damaged, and the brain had no ability to regenerate. These old concepts are being challenged by new science. There is now increasing evidence that rehabilitation can actually drive brain reorganization to allow previously dormant or under-used regions to take over functions damaged by the stroke. Imaging studies have demonstrated that new regions 'light up' as function improves. This has rejuvenated rehabilitation as there is now good reason to believe that newer rehabilitation techniques and intensity could drive better recovery from stroke. This fits in with what many patients tell us: motivated patients who really work hard at rehabilitation and training after stroke can sometimes achieve remarkable recoveries. This is called **brain plasticity**, and the new concept of rehabilitation is to take advantage of this and focus more research on getting better and earlier recovery after stroke.

 Patient's perspective

Ross Pearson was 40 years old when he had his stroke in January 2000 whilst cycling with his wife on a training ride in the local park. His symptoms started with pins and needles down the right side of his body, and shortly afterwards he collapsed and was taken to hospital. He awoke 3 days later in the intensive care unit and was told that he had had a primary intracerebral haemorrhage stroke affecting his left brain which had caused a severe right-sided weakness, aphasia, loss of the right visual field, and complete loss of sensation down the right side. After 4 months of hospital rehabilitation he was discharged home with a wheelchair, but was able to walk around the house. He decided to hire a personal trainer for daily training in addition to the twice weekly outpatient hospital rehabilitation. A year later he was walking, swimming 1 km three times a week, and achieved his goal of riding his bicycle again. In 2005 he and his wife cycled 19 000 km around Australia on a tandem. In 2007 he enjoys work, and still thinks he is improving. He is a Stroke Ambassador for the Australian National Stroke Foundation.

Physiotherapy

What rehabilitation methods work best?

This is a really interesting question and one brought forcefully to my attention when I moved from the UK to Australia to work as I also moved from a stroke rehabilitation environment dominated by Bobath-trained physiotherapists to an Australian environment dominated by evidence-based medicine physiotherapy schools who taught a Movement Science (or Motor Relearning) method (see box). What happened to my patients? Well, I must admit that despite the two very different methods, I did not really notice a great deal of difference in their recovery. However, I was aware of a lot more 'training' in Australia, and less work done on a plinth or static work in a gym. In practice, it is quite difficult to perform comparative studies. One reason is that physiotherapists have strong views on which method is effective and questioning this view is not popular! However, several comparisons have been made with differing results, although the Motor Relearning approach has either been as effective as or superior to other methods in the studies to date. With the new emphasis on evidence-based medicine, it is likely that Motor Relearning will become increasingly dominant, but clinical practice will take time to change. However, I believe that Bobath therapists now have a responsibility to evaluate their methods against the newer work of Carr and Shepherd.

Physiotherapy methods

Bobath method

This physiotherapy method was developed by Berta Bobath (1907–1991), a physiotherapist, and her husband, who was medically qualified and trained in paediatrics. They fled from Germany before the Second World War and developed their style of physiotherapy in London in the post-war years.

The Bobath method is also described as a neurodevelopmental method and, in brief, has a framework of improving patients with stroke by a very hands-on approach with the major aim of normalizing muscle tone (e.g. reducing spasticity) and movement patterns. This method has become the dominant approach in the UK and Europe and has become an oral tradition taught by experts. One aspect of this approach which is particularly relevant is that therapists often purposefully delay task specific movements (e.g. walking) if they fear that this will reinforce abnormal patterns of movement. This approach has particularly been used for children with cerebral palsy.

Movement Science (Motor Relearning)

This approach has been led by Janet Carr and Roberta Shepherd, senior academic physiotherapists at the University of Sydney. It is very much a scientific method, based on the movement sciences with a large evidence base supporting effectiveness. This approach uses context-specific functional training as the mainstay of therapy. In other words, if the person with stroke has a weak leg, this approach uses training to improve strength and walking practice to improve gait.

Comment

I have found that physiotherapists generally put great faith in their particular style of practice and any questioning of their particular method can evoke reactions as if questioning someone's religious beliefs! However, it must be said that many therapists use an eclectic mix of the Bobath and Motor Relearning methods which, over time, they have found to be effective.

Some additional observations on physiotherapy approaches

In the Stroke Unit Trials overview (see Chapter 5, Cochrane Library), one of the best results came from the Trondheim unit in Norway. At this stroke unit at St Olav's University Hospital, their emphasis is on a very early functional and intense approach to mobilization with the physiotherapists working with the nursing staff, so that every aspect of care becomes an opportunity for training. Whilst this style of physiotherapy is unusual, the excellent results from this unit have prompted further research on very early and intense training.

The Motor Relearning approach is also very dependent on active involvement by patients, and as dementia and cognitive impairment are quite common in people with stroke, there may be advantages of using a Bobath approach which is much more of a hands-on therapy. This might be a more useful technique for the more passive patients.

Intensity

Although the approaches to physiotherapy may be controversial, we are on safer ground when discussing how much therapy should be given. There is evidence that more therapy is better than less, and this certainly would fit with our new ideas of brain plasticity. Many patients with stroke, even on stroke units, spend the majority of their time resting, and therefore there is great scope for improving physiotherapy time which should lead to better outcomes. People with stroke can tolerate additional sessions without excessive fatigue.

Medical care

The medical issues in the acute phase concern accurate diagnosis, assessment, and treatment. In the weeks following stroke, medical care and rehabilitation is the mainstay of care, and rehabilitation and general practice take over in the months following stroke. These phases need different skills, and different models of care have evolved. It probably does not matter which medical speciality provides stroke unit care (general internal medicine, geriatric medicine, or neurology) provided that the physicians have appropriate stroke training. If neurologists or internists provide the day-to-day care for acute stroke units, there is often transfer of care to rehabilitation units for those requiring prolonged rehabilitation. Geriatricians may be able to offer continuity of care in the rehabilitation setting. Given that stroke is increasingly a disease of the frail elderly, it is important that all stroke doctors maintain general medical skills as patients with stroke commonly have other problems in the acute phase. The types of medical problems and complications seen in the acute phase of stroke are shown in Table 6.1.

In Table 6.1 it can be seen that the proportion of people with stroke having seizures (epileptic fits) remains low at about 5 per cent. However, it is important to note that stroke becomes the main cause of new seizures in old age. Seizures can occur at stroke onset (about 1 in 50), and it is important not to attribute stroke as the cause until stroke mimics (cerebral tumour or abscess, or encephalitis) or other common precipitants (alcohol withdrawal, drugs, metabolic causes) have been ruled out. A further complication is that

Table 6.1 Complications and medical problems after stroke

Complication/medical problem	Frequency after stroke
In the first few weeks	
Heart rhythm disturbances (e.g. AF)	10–20%
Worsening of stroke	20–50%
Recurrent stroke	2–5%
Heart attack	1%
Gastrointestinal bleeding	3%
Pneumonia	10–20%
Urinary tract infections	25%
Other infections	10%
Urinary incontinence	50%
Faecal incontinence	25%
Pressure sores	<5%*
Deep vein thrombosis	5–25%†
Pulmonary embolism	1–2%
High blood sugar (hyperglycaemia)	40%
Pain (multifactorial)	30%
Falls	20–30%
Fractures	2–5%
In the first year of stroke	
Seizures	5%
Depression	25%
Central post-stroke pain	5%
Dementia	10–20%
Emotionalism	15%
Anxiety	20%

*Pressure sores are easily preventable, and units should strive to get these complications as low as possible.
†The rate of deep vein thrombosis is highly dependent on what test is used to detect them.

some seizures can mimic stroke – a syndrome called Todd's paresis. Treatment of the initial seizure may be required if it is prolonged, and treatment to prevent further seizures will depend on several factors such as whether there have been recurrent attacks, or if a further seizure would have major implications for the patient (e.g. removal of driving licence).

The role of the medical staff on the stroke unit, in addition to their medical duties described above, will usually include managing the unit and leading multidisciplinary team meetings. One component of an effective stroke unit is continued professional training, and the medical staff have an important role to play in teaching both medical staff and other healthcare professionals.

Nursing

As with physiotherapy, there are a number of different nursing styles (team nursing, primary nursing, etc.), but there are limited data on the effectiveness of these styles in stroke medicine. Stroke nursing should be considered a nursing speciality in the same way as cardiac nursing or intensive care nursing. Nursing staff have a particularly important role in stroke medicine, given that many patients with stroke need nursing staff to provide all their care needs. Many nursing issues will be dealt with in the section on complications after stroke, but some of the more important aspects of stroke nursing care include:

- provision of activities of daily living:
    - bathing
    - toileting
    - grooming
    - eating
    - continence

- comfort care

- positioning and facilitating movement and training

- hydration and care of intravenous treatment

- information and support

- deep venous thrombosis prophylaxis

♦ palliation for those who are terminally ill

♦ giving medication.

Speech therapy/speech pathology

The healthcare professional specializing in speech problems after stroke is called a speech and language therapist (or speech pathologist in many countries). Their role in stroke has evolved to encompass not only the assessment and treatment of language problems but also swallowing problems (dysphagia). There is often a shortage of such staff, and in some stroke units the nursing staff assess swallowing problems. The shortage of staff can also lead to a situation where the therapists merely assess the problems and cannot provide therapy, which is unfortunate as there is now good evidence that regular speech therapy can improve the outcome after stroke (with respect to brain plasticity and training). Therapy (training) should begin without delay after stroke (ideally the next working day), and involve sessions of 1–2 hours a day. There is evidence that the help of others (e.g. volunteers), group work, and computer-based therapy are all effective. There is uncertainty about the use of specific medication (e.g. stimulants such as amphetamines, or other treatments such as piracetam) as none of the randomized controlled trials have been large enough to establish effectiveness and none have been able to exclude an important hazard such as increasing the death rate! The actual content of speech therapy is beyond the remit of this book, but there is evidence that phonetic and semantic training is effective.

Evidence from 'before and after' studies have conclusively shown that checking a person's swallowing function before allowing them to eat reduces aspiration. Speech therapists will guide stroke unit staff in the correct diet to be used (see box page 88). Objective evidence of dysphagia can be obtained by using a special X-ray technique (Modified Barium Swallow) where a radiodense substance (e.g. barium) is swallowed and monitored by a X-ray image intensifier supervised by the radiologist and speech therapist. This can be helpful in uncertain cases although the exact role for this invasive test has yet to be established.

Dietary modification after stroke

Instruction	Rationale
Nil by mouth	People should not eat or drink after a stroke until their swallowing has been tested
Thickened fluids	A special thickener is used to make liquids safe to swallow for people with dysphagia
Thickened fluids and puree diet	Food is introduced in puree form
Normal diet with supervision	Supervision may be required to remind people to eat slowly and swallow carefully
Normal diet	When dysphagia resolves

Occupational therapy

The role of the occupational therapist varies from country to country. In some countries, there are no occupational therapists in stroke units and their role is taken on by nursing staff or physiotherapists. In the UK (and Australia) the role of the occupational therapist includes the assessment of basic and more advanced functional activities. In medical terminology, the basic activities required to exist in a reasonable state are called **activities of daily living,** and more advanced activities are referred to as **extended activities of daily living** (see box).

Activities of daily living (ADLs) and extended (instrumental) activities of daily living (EADLs)

ADLs

Bathing, and use of shower or bath

Mobility (walking on the flat and stairs)

Continence (bladder and bowel)

Toileting

Grooming (e.g. combing hair, shaving)

Dressing

Feeding

The ability to accomplish these basic ADLs is usually a requirement for return home.

Extended ADLs

Cooking

Shopping

Leisure activities

Driving a car

Riding a bicycle

Using public transport

Getting out in the community

The ability to accomplish extended ADLs usually adds enormously to quality of life

Impairments that impact on ADLs and EADLs

Dementia and cognitive impairment can have a huge effect on the person's ability to complete these activities. Many people with such problems may manage these tasks only with supervision.

Aphasia

Problems with language may not affect ADLs but have a huge effect on EADLs (e.g. the ability to ask for shopping items)

Postscript

A recent study identified that being able to shop is currently the most sought after EADL for stroke survivors!

The occupational therapist will work on specific tasks in collaboration with nursing staff and physiotherapists. This will involve a period of assessment, including the ability to understand instructions (commonly disrupted by aphasia and dementia), followed by specific training in basic ADLs. For example, when patients have enough motor recovery to maintain sitting balance, it is possible to start working on basic washing (e.g. washing the face, cleaning the teeth). As recovery proceeds, more complex tasks can be assessed and practised (e.g. getting on and off the toilet, getting dressed, and feeding).

The occupational therapist has a very important role in predicting how people will manage at home, and when there is doubt, or after a particularly severe stroke, they will often (together with other members of the stroke team) perform a home visit, with or without the patient, to determine how feasible discharge home will be.

Social work

Again, the requirement for social workers will depend on the make-up of society. In societies with no social support systems a social worker will be of little use! In the UK and many European countries, there is an often bewildering collection of services for the person with stroke. This can range from a home help who can do the shopping and clean the house, to a full package of domiciliary care to get someone out of bed, washed, dressed, and toileted, the reverse at night, and all meals (called the dawn and dusk visits plus meals). This all costs money, and social workers are essential to help navigate through the myriad of services and regulations. They are particularly important if, as commonly occurs, the patient is unlikely to recover well enough to return home and alternative arrangements are required, such as a nursing home or supported accommodation.

Clinical psychology

Psychologists can have an important role to play in stroke units. Their expertise may be particularly useful in assessing mood and depression, helping people through difficult adjustment periods, managing difficult behaviour and other distress, and providing cognitive therapy. Cognitive therapy is a behavioural technique which is used to help stroke patients recover, and covers areas such as concentration, attention, orientation to time and day, and memory. At present, there is a limited evidence base for such techniques, but improvements in cognitive scales and measures have been shown by interventions delivered by clinical psychologists and, in keeping with the theme of brain plasticity, it is highly likely that this type of training technique will help people recover from stroke. However, there are some provisos. Research has struggled to find treatments that make a difference in overall activities or disability level, people need to be able to tolerate the treatments (and many people with stroke will not because of dementia, drowsiness, or fatigue), and clinical psychologists are few and far between in most stroke services. It is very possible that other members of the stroke team can take on some of these roles, but this will depend on the complexity of the technique used.

Dietetics

Dieticians should play a role in a stroke unit. Some people are so dysphagic that they have to be tube fed, and such feeding requires an appropriate liquid feed, commenced at the appropriate rate and monitored carefully. If patients are tube fed after a period of starvation, there is a 'refeeding syndrome' that can be dangerous, and appropriate precautions must be taken to avoid this. In the recovery period after stroke, people should be advised to adopt a healthy diet, low in salt and saturated fats, with plenty of fresh fruit and vegetables, and dieticians can help counsel patients and their families.

Pharmacy

Pharmacists have a crucial role to play in many hospital services, especially the stroke service. The use of medication is such a complex area that it is renowned for causing a large number of hospital errors. Any help in reducing these errors is welcome. Medication use has become very important in stroke medicine, as numerous randomized controlled trials have established the use of a variety of different treatments not only to treat the stroke itself, but also to ward off another stroke (see Chapter 8). In addition, many patients with stroke have swallowing difficulties, and sometimes medication may be given by the intravenous route, or rectally by suppository, or crushed down a feeding tube, and pharmacists can advise on these matters.

The family

The family and/or the patient's carer has a crucial role to play after a stroke. Their support will usually be of great comfort for the patient, and when the stroke has caused major problems, their help in the recovery process is a key part of good stroke unit care. This can include getting the family to reinforce particular training sessions and training family members to manage the patient with a view to discharge (e.g. teaching techniques to transfer the patient from bed to wheelchair, or getting the patient into a car safely). Families also need information about stroke in general and about the progress of the patient.

Team work

A good stroke team will work seamlessly with the patient and their family, and help the patient achieve realistic goals in their stroke journey. This will need regular meetings (at least weekly), and it is important that the team is flexible as many events can upset the predicted course (see Fig. 6.1 and Table 6.1). These can be patient related (e.g. they have an early recurrent stroke or other major medical illness), family related (e.g. the main carer at home comes to the conclusion that it would be too difficult to look after the patient because of their stroke problems), environment related (e.g. social support services are unavailable), or a dispute between the healthcare team and the family (e.g. the family are convinced that the patient needs more time in rehabilitation, but the team believe that there is no prospect of meaningful recovery).

If the stroke patient is in a hospital stroke unit, the most optimistic goal is discharge back home from the unit, and the majority of people admitted to hospital with stroke will return home (about 60 per cent). This discharge plan is obvious for those with non-disabling stroke, and can be reasonably predicted for many others (e.g. for those rapidly improving). Sadly, for others it is often apparent that the stroke will be a fatal event and palliative care is appropriate. In a substantial minority of patients, there will be uncertainty; their stroke will be disabling, and for all sorts of reasons the future cannot be easily predicted. The best course of action is to see what happens with a reasonable trial of rehabilitation; the likely future often becomes obvious. If the patient remains very dependent after several weeks of rehabilitation, the decision whether to continue or not will depend on many factors: younger patients often have more potential for slow sustained recovery; those with other medical illnesses (comorbidity) are likely to fare less well; those who are slowly improving are worth persevering with; those with an obvious treatable cause of a slow recovery may need more time (e.g. patients who have become profoundly depressed need treatment of the depression); for the others, it is best to plan for future care at their current level of abilities.

Discharge planning

Discharge planning has many experts but little hard evidence, and the consensus is that we often do it badly! This is a complex area, and much can go wrong. The ideal discharge from hospital should be viewed as a transfer of care to a community team to continue the good work, whether this is appropriate medical supervision for the patient with a non-disabling stroke or transfer to a community stroke rehabilitation team to continue active therapy for several more weeks. Most complaints arise because key people (e.g. the family doctor, the family, the home help, or the hospital transport service) are not kept fully informed.

In many areas, rehabilitation is continued in the community, as early supported discharge services have been shown to be effective at reducing length of hospital stays with similar results to hospital stroke units. These teams usually include physiotherapists and occupational therapists, augmented by nurses and speech therapists. The provision of social care and 24-hour care will facilitate even earlier discharge from hospital. These services have generally been shown to be similar in cost to hospital care; they are usually well received by patients but at a cost of increased stress for the carers.

Despite how well transfer of care is organized, many people with stroke feel very isolated and unsupported following discharge from hospital. The issues that affect people after stroke is the topic for the next chapter.

Further reading

Australian National Stroke Foundation (2005) *Clinical Guidelines for Stroke Rehabilitation and Recovery. Approved by the National Health & Medical Research Council of Australia.* Available online at: www.strokefoundation.com.au

Langhorne P, Stott DJ, Robertson L, *et al.* (2000) Medical complications after stroke: a multicentre study. *Stroke*, **31**, 1223–9.

Davenport RJ, Dennis MS, Wellwood I, and Warlow CP (1996). Complications after acute stroke. *Stroke*, **27**, 415–20.

7

Living after stroke

 Key points

◆ Patients living with stroke need access to appropriate advice.

◆ Depression, memory problems and pain are examples of post-stroke problems that need to be addressed.

◆ Support for carers is important and provision of respite care will help many severely disabled stroke survivors remain at home.

Living after stroke presents numerous different challenges as people are so different from each other, and strokes can vary from the trivial to the devastating. Every stroke survivor will have a different story and differing problems and challenges to overcome, and this chapter cannot do much more than discuss some common issues. Research in this area has found that some 'obvious' solutions are no solutions at all! For example, provision of some types of support can make stroke survivors more helpless! The key appears to be to enable people to solve their own problems – easier said than done.

Common early problems

Difficulty swallowing

Up to half of all people with stroke will have difficulty swallowing food or water in the first few days and weeks following their stroke, a problem called **dysphagia**. One immediate consequence of this is that no one should eat or drink after a stroke until their swallowing ability has been checked. Fortunately, in most people swallowing function returns during the early rehabilitation phase.

Recent research has also clarified the role of feeding for patients with stroke. First, if the patient is reasonably nourished and able to swallow safely, there is no major benefit in using additional feeding supplements in the recovery phase of stroke (it had been thought that supplements would benefit patients in this critical time period). If the patient is unable to swallow in the first week after the stroke, early tube feeding does not lead to an increase in independent survival, but may reduce deaths. Unfortunately, people 'saved' by early tube feeding remain very disabled. This is probably because if dysphagia is present, it is likely to have been caused by a major stroke, and the other consequences of this sort of stroke overwhelm the theoretical benefits of early feeding. A feeding tube is not a trivial intervention: it can be uncomfortable and unsightly, and appears to cause bleeding in the gut in some people. Therefore a decision to use tube feeding early after stroke needs to be an individual one, made after discussion with the patient and family. Patients often have firm views on this, and it is not uncommon for families to report: 'Mother said she would never want to be kept alive with tube feeding'. If swallowing remains impaired and a decision is made to tube feed the patient, there are two main tube options: a tube placed in the stomach through the nose (nasogastric tube) or a tube placed in an endoscopic technique through the stomach wall called a percutaneous endoscopically placed gastroenterostomy (PEG) tube. Research has shown that the use of a nasogastric tube in the first few weeks of dysphagic stroke is more likely to be associated with eating normally at 6 months and has a marginal benefit in terms of quality of life. However, the trials also demonstrated that this problem is usually associated with very severe strokes indeed, and quality of life is likely to remain very poor despite every effort to improve feeding. If long-term tube feeding is required, a PEG tube is the only practical option.

Incontinence

Incontinence of urine and faeces is very common after stroke, and there has been very little investigation of the best way to manage it, possibly because the subject is a rather unglamorous complication of a poorly funded disease! Despite the paucity of good data to guide management, there is general consensus about a few matters.

◆ Continence care should be a priority in the stroke unit.

◆ Urinary catheters should be avoided unless absolutely necessary.

◆ Modern technology such as bedside ultrasound scanners ('bladder scanners') has revolutionized the detection of incomplete bladder emptying and will help guide management.

◆ Intermittent catheterization may avoid the need for a permanent catheter in some patients.

◆ Regular toileting and avoidance of constipation will help bowel care.

◆ Ward-based protocols can help improve continence care.

If continence cannot be achieved, urinary catheterization and appropriate provision of continence care pads may be required. Faecal incontinence may be particularly distressing, and sometimes a regimen of using a constipating agent and regular enemas may achieve faecal continence for some people requiring high-level nursing care.

Tiredness

Many people find that they become very tired after having a stroke. This is actually a common problem after any major illness. It is important to ensure that the tiredness is not due to a medical problem such as anaemia or a psychological cause such as depression. In the absence of an obvious medical cause, a graduated increase in exercise may help.

Depression

Stroke comes as a great shock to most people, and it is very understandable when people become upset and miserable after such an event. However, in a proportion of people this reaction becomes severe and the features of depression become prominent. Depression is a major complication of stroke and affects about a fifth of stroke survivors in the first year after stroke. When depression arises in the early phase of the post-stroke recovery it can manifest in many different ways, and it is often the therapists and nurses who notice the changes first. Physiotherapists report poor concentration, or perhaps a 'failure to thrive', i.e. a lack of progress in an expected recovery. For many reasons it can be challenging to diagnose a depressive illness after stroke: the stroke may have caused aphasia, with a resulting difficulty in communication; speech may have become monotonous ('depressed') because of damage to the right side of the brain; sleep patterns may have altered become of the stroke and not necessarily because of depression; frequent crying may actually be due to 'emotionalism' rather than a depressive problem. Because of these difficulties, a psychiatric assessment may be useful. Rather surprisingly, there have been few well-designed studies of the best way to treat depression in stroke patients, and we are dependent on using data from other situations. We know that antidepressants are generally effective for older people with other medical problems and for people with depression who are otherwise well. Therefore, in the absence of good stroke studies, antidepressants are used when depression has been diagnosed. In keeping with practice for non-stroke patients, treatment is often required for a considerable time (e.g. 9–12 months), with perhaps a gradual reduction after that time if the person has remained well. Cognitive behavioural therapy is not proven in this situation but behavioural therapies may help. Experts in the field recognize that the evidence base in this area is poor and more research is required for such a common problem.

Given its high prevalence, there has been great interest in trying to prevent depression and three interventions show promise: stroke unit care, problem-solving therapy, and motivational interviewing. The last two interventions emphasize the importance of the person taking control of their lives in order to improve their emotional well-being, and both imply that the person needs to invest time and energy into strategies to improve their quality of life. Taking a pill is often not the best answer to a problem!

Common later problems

Pain

Pain is not usually the first symptom you think about when considering stroke, but it can occur. Many strokes are associated with pain; for example, primary intracerebral haemorrhage commonly occurs with sudden headache. The onset of ischaemic stroke can also be associated with pain which localizes to the side of the stroke lesion (usually opposite the side of the body affected by the stroke). This type of stroke-onset pain usually resolves over the following hours and days. However, the disability of stroke can result in different causes of pain. In the acute hospital phase of stroke a variety of tubes are required to maintain life and manage the acute problems, and these may be uncomfortable. Some of the complications of disability (e.g. pressure sores and deep vein thromboses), now readily preventable and so hopefully seen only rarely, can be painful. Complications of the paralysis of stroke can lead to a painful shoulder, but this again is readily preventable with the best rehabilitation practice. It must not be forgotten that many people with stroke will have had potentially painful conditions before their stroke, and these conditions (e.g. arthritis and gout) may be made worse by the stroke.

Central pain can be caused by stroke (and also by a long list of other neurological conditions). This type of pain has many other names (see box page 99) and is caused by damage to parts of the brain involved in the processing of pain and the normal pain pathways. The thalamus is particularly important area for pain processing, so that strokes in and around this region are more likely to be associated with the central pain syndrome.

Alternative names for the central pain syndrome

- Thalamic pain syndrome

- Central post-stroke syndrome

- Dejerine–Roussy syndrome

- Retrolenticular syndrome

- Neuropathic pain

- Posterior thalamic syndrome

Central pain after stroke can occur immediately after the stroke but may often have delayed onset for some weeks or months. About 2–8 per cent of people with stroke will have central post-stroke pain. Patients use a large variety of different descriptions for the pain, including like tooth-ache, searing, deep burning, stretching, tightness, itching, steady, continuous – all clearly unpleasant sensations. The pain tends to affect areas of the body affected by weakness, and a person who has a weak left arm and leg may experience central pain in the left arm and leg. Characteristically, the pain is made worse by touching the affected area, and a light touch may be felt as a very different sensation. This condition is called **dysaesthesia**. Once recognized as central pain, the key aspects of treatment are explanation and appropriate painkillers. For example, patients are reassured that the pain is not a warning of another stroke. Painkillers such as paracetamol and ibuprofen are often ineffective, and randomized controlled trials have identified that other treatments such as amitriptyline (an older antidepressant) and carbamazepine (an anticonvulsant) are effective.

Memory and cognitive problems

As stroke is characterized by damage to part of the brain it is inevitable that certain strokes will cause damage to memory and other aspects of cognition. **Cognition** is the name given to the mental functions carried out by the human brain, including comprehension and use of speech, visual perception and construction, calculation ability, attention (information processing), memory, and executive functions such as planning, problem-solving, and self-monitoring. Memory problems are very common, and for some merely represent a reaction to the shock of having a stroke. However, for others, stroke causes a sudden loss of function which it never regains, and as such stroke is the second most important cause of dementia (after Alzheimer's disease). During the first few hours and days of stroke, the assessments of cognitive ability usually include assessment of speech function (see Chapter 6) and screening for memory problems. As people recover, it may become necessary to assess cognitive function in greater detail. This is particularly important for those still in work, those who are experiencing major problems such as depression or anger, or those who rely on particular skills such as driving. In this situation it can be useful to consult a clinical psychologist who can assess mental function in great detail and advise on strategies to cope with any identified problems. Unfortunately, we do not have a great repertoire of treatments that are definitely of benefit in this area – this is yet another area of stroke medicine requiring considerable more research. However, cognitive treatments that have been shown to have some benefit or value are shown in the box. It should be noted that these treatments and interventions do not necessarily need to be delivered by psychologists; some may be best done by occupational therapists or even family members or carers themselves. In general, practice can often improve abilities, and families, friends, and carers can all help by encouraging people who have had a stroke to practise their memory, attention span, and more complex mental abilities.

Beneficial treatments or interventions for cognitive problems after stroke

◆ Cognitive rehabilitation to improve attention

◆ External cues to prompt memory

◆ Devices (e.g. pagers) to initiate everyday activities

◆ Computer-based training to improve visual function

◆ Scanning training to improve neglect

Driving after stroke

There are two main issues to consider. Has the patient made a sufficient physical and cognitive recovery to be able to drive? Do the local legal requirements allow patients to drive? Some people with minor stroke may be perfectly competent to drive but legally unable to do so. The legal restrictions vary from country to country. In the UK, for example, people are not allowed to drive for 1 month after a stroke or TIA. Patients should only return to driving after checking the current legal and insurance rules that apply and on the advice of their doctor. Certain stroke deficits will result in a permanent driving ban such as hemianopia (loss of one visual field) and certain physical impairments will make driving impossible. When there is doubt, or for reassurance, there are special occupational therapy driving units that are able to assess driving skills off the road and to perform on the road tests.

Sex after stroke

 Case study

I am reminded of a patient of mine when I was a junior doctor. I was working in a geriatric day hospital, and one of the attendees certainly was not a geriatric patient in age, being only in her fifties. However, she had a severe hemiparesis, was wheelchair bound, and had a urinary catheter. I had to see her one day because she wanted to try and manage without her urinary catheter. This had been a major problem as she suffered from terrible urinary incontinence without the catheter; however, she was insistent that it was removed. The nurses and I were equally insistent that it was the best solution to a difficult problem. Eventually, she told me that the real reason she wanted to have the catheter removed was that it interfered with her ability to have satisfactory sex with her husband. I learnt an important lesson! Despite the natural reserve many people have in talking about sexual behaviour, it is sometimes important to discuss these private and delicate matters.

If sex was an important part of life before a stroke, it is likely that this will be the case afterwards. Stroke will have several major effects on sexual function. The psychological aspects of stroke may affect confidence and lead to an inability to sustain an erection. Sex drive may disappear for quite a while in some, but in others the opportunities of being close to a partner may actually increase sexual desire. The physical limitations of the stroke (e.g. arm and leg weakness) may limit previous sexual athleticism. Incontinence issues may lead to urinary catheterization which could potentially limit intercourse. Aphasia may lead to great difficulties in communication with the inevitable effect on intimacy and perhaps foreplay. Medication (e.g. some antihypertensives) may contribute to male impotence or vaginal dryness.

The changing roles of a spouse, perhaps in becoming a major carer, can affect relationships, and of course this can go both ways. Many people worry about the risks of having another stroke during sex but the risks are probably the same as having a further stroke whilst exercising. Both these occurrences are rare but can occur. Worries of this type should be discussed with partners and healthcare staff. In fact, talking about these issues with partners is of great importance, and there are many general interventions that may help improve sex after stroke, or encourage resumption of usual activity. These include the importance of physical contact, taking things slowly and gently at first, avoiding excessive alcohol, adjusting medication if impotence is medication related, using lubricants if dryness is an issue, experimenting with other forms of intimacy (e.g. mutual masturbation rather than intercourse), taping urinary catheter tubing out of the way, or relying on intermittent catherization (females), doubling back catheter tubing and the penis and catheter tubing with a condom for males, and ensuring appropriate hygiene and cleanliness to improve self-esteem and attractiveness.

Occasionally, the stroke can cause disinhibition or hypersexuality. If this is a problem, it should be recognized as being a complication or reaction to the stroke and may require assessment and treatment.

Women of childbearing age must not assume that the stroke will render them infertile! As the oral contraceptive pill can increase the risk of stroke, alternative methods (e.g. barrier contraception, vasectomy of partner) should be considered, and this may be something to discuss with the general practitioner.

Support after stroke

Patients, their carers, and their families need appropriate support after stroke. However, it is not always easy to know what support is most useful. For example, one randomized controlled trial of a stroke family support officer found evidence of survivors of stroke becoming more helpless if provided with a support officer. The main themes arising from this and other research is that people need to be supported to solve problems themselves, and not just be given pre-prepared solutions to common problems. However, there are some very practical issues that need to be addressed, and sadly this often does not happen. If the stroke has caused severe disability and care is being provided at home, usually by one main carer, it is important to support that carer with services such as in-home respite which allows him/her to go out for some hours for a break, or maybe to do some of the essential activities of life such as shopping. Some carers need more prolonged respite and find that regular respite care is an essential part of the long-term plan. Services vary widely, but commonly stroke patients can be provided with temporary care in a residential facility to help the main carer have a holiday, recover from an illness, or simply have a break.

In many areas there are services to help with the care of people at home. These can include help with domestic work, personal care of the person with stroke, and sometimes more skilled nursing care.

 Case study

A seventy year old lady had a severe stroke affecting her left face, arm, and leg. She also had marked inattention to her left hand side which made rehabilitation slow going. Due to nursing home shortages at that particular time, she spent many months in the rehabilitation ward and during the stay she got some friends to bring in some pictures of her beloved bungalow and garden. Her garden was absolutely beautiful and her clear love of her home was a helpful additional incentive for the stroke team to work even harder to be able to get her home. Eventually she did indeed go home, initially supported by a maximum home care package which consisted of a 'dawn' service to help her get out of bed, get washed, and have breakfast. Carers came in at lunch time to help her prepare a meal, and in the evening she had the 'dusk' service to ensure she had eaten her evening meal and to help her get into bed. She was wheelchair independent and was overjoyed about living at home. Interestingly, this was one of my Scottish patients. Australia is about 10 years behind in the ageing demographics and also home services and I cannot currently get such a package of care for my Sydney patients, but I suspect this will come eventually.

The leading stroke charities find that a very important aspect of their care is providing a help-line service for advice. Carers often comment to me that the ability to talk to someone about their problems and pressures can be very helpful and routine health professionals (e.g. general practitioners and practice nurses) have an important role in this. Some information about helplines is given in the appendix.

Spasticity

Spasticity is the increase in tone during muscle movement and is one of the features of the physiological changes that occur after a stroke. My observation is that troublesome spasticity is less of a problem when patients have appropriate early rehabilitation and stroke unit care. It is often a particularly difficult problem if, for example, a younger patient has required care in the intensive care unit for several weeks because of a very severe stroke. In this situation, only passive movements are possible, and when active rehabilitation commences the therapists often need to spend a considerable amount of time trying to reduce the spasticity which is now causing spasms, flexion contractures, and limitations of movement.

Spasticity affecting the fingers can in time lead to the fist closing up, which can prevent basic hygiene and also severely affect function. In this situation some practitioners use botulinum toxin to reduce the tone (of course, this will make the muscles even weaker). Prevention is better than cure and physical therapy with passive and active stretching through the whole motion of the affected limb is part of the physiotherapist's repertoire of interventions after stroke.

Further reading

Australian National Stroke Foundation (2005) *Clinical Guidelines for Stroke Rehabilitation and Recovery*. Approved by the National Health & Medical. Australian National Stroke Foundation. Available online at http://www.strokefoundation.com.au

UK National Clinical Guidelines for Stroke: available online at http://www.rcplondon.ac.uk/pubs/books/stroke/

8

How do you
prevent stroke?

⟳ Key points

♦ Lifestyle changes to reduce dietary salt and cholesterol, together with a reduction in cigarette smoking, will lead to a large drop in stroke incidence.

♦ Lifestyle changes plus medication are required for certain high-risk patients.

♦ Following a stroke, lifestyle changes, medication, and possibly surgery are required to reduce the change of further strokes and other vascular diseases.

The important lesson about stroke prevention is that we know what causes the majority of strokes and we know how to prevent stroke. The challenge is being able to apply that knowledge in a feasible and affordable manner worldwide. In medical terms prevention is usually split into primary and secondary prevention. The differences are important: primary prevention refers to efforts to prevent stroke in people (or a population) who have not had a stroke, whereas secondary prevention aims to prevent a second, or subsequent, stroke. It is also important to note that the term 'stroke' also includes transient ischaemic attack (TIA), as the risks of future strokes (or other problems such as heart attacks) are more or less the same for both. The reason that prevention is usually split into 'primary' and 'secondary' prevention is that the risks of stroke are very different in these two situations; in fact, the risk of stroke in stroke survivors is approximately 10 times that of someone who has never had a stroke. This substantial increase in the risk of future stroke means that secondary preventative measures are generally more cost effective (the 'number needed to treat' is less), but also allows us to consider more risky preventative strategies (a higher potential benefit is worth the higher potential risk). Conversely, **primary** preventative strategies need to be 10 times **safer** if they are to have net benefit. Preventative strategies are always a balance of risks and benefits of the strategy under question. If the benefits are greater for people who have already had a stroke, riskier strategies can be, and are, considered. Stroke preventative strategies for healthy people have to be extremely safe as more people will be exposed to the potential risks for a given (smaller) benefit.

Another important factor to consider is the cause of stroke. Although most strokes are due to the complications of atheroma, a minority of strokes are due to one-off defined reasons. Secondary prevention of this type of event depends on the cause. For example, if the stroke was due to vasculitis, control of the vasculitis will be the best long-term strategy. If the stroke is thought to be due to tight carotid stenosis, then prompt surgery is the key to prevention (in addition to vascular secondary preventative measures). This issue is particularly relevant for paediatric stroke as these strokes are *not* due to the complications of atheroma or life-long hypertension. The secondary prevention of further stroke in children crucially depends on correctly identifying the cause and treating this. For example, if the stroke is due to sickle cell anaemia there is now good evidence that transfusion to maintain the abnormal sickle haemoglobin (HbS) below 30 per cent will prevent further ischaemic strokes. Stroke in the neonatal period is usually due to complications of the neonatal period, and thus this group of infants have a very low risk of recurrent stroke. In older children it is important to treat the cause (e.g. treatment of vasculitis) but, reassuringly, if investigations show no abnormality in the blood vessels the risk of recurrence is low.

The new guidelines on vascular disease prevention (which of course includes stroke) make the primary and secondary split rather artificial as strategies are being recommended after estimating individual risk, and vascular disease is so common that there are many people who are now considered high risk but who do not have symptoms. In addition, it is artificial to concentrate only on stroke prevention, as people with stroke are also at high risk of the other common vascular diseases such as heart attack, peripheral vascular disease, and sudden death. Therefore it is now best to include stroke prevention as part of vascular prevention and to consider three distinct categories of people: low-risk asymptomatic individuals (i.e. those who have never had a stroke), high-risk asymptomatic individuals, and symptomatic individuals (those who have had a stroke or TIA). In general, lifestyle changes are best for low-risk asymptomatic individuals, lifestyle changes and medication are recommended for high-risk asymptomatic individuals, and secondary prevention usually entails multiple medication and lifestyle changes plus some surgical approaches for a few individuals.

High risk is currently arbitrarily defined as a 20 per cent risk of a stroke, heart attack, or other serious vascular event in the next 10 years, but this definition is more to do with affordability and cost-effectiveness than any other reason. If you are worried about stroke or want to estimate your vascular risk, there are freely available internet calculators (web sites listed in the appendix). Examples of typical 10-year risks are shown in the box.

Estimated vascular risks

Less than 10 per cent chance of vascular event in 10 years

- 43 years old, male, non-smoker, total cholesterol 5.0 mmol/litre, BP 120/80

- 43 years old, male, smoker, total cholesterol 5 mmol/litre, BP 120/80★

- 43 years old, female, non-smoker, total cholesterol 6.0 mmol/litre, BP 160/80

20 per cent risk of vascular event in 10 years (i.e. threshold of 'high-risk' asymptomatic individual)

- 43 years old, male, smoker, total cholesterol 5 mmol/litre, BP 180/90

- 43 years old female, smoker, total cholesterol 8.0 mmol/litre, BP 180/90†

- 73 years old, male, non-smoker, total cholesterol 5.0 mmol/litre, BP 120/80†

- 73 years old, female, smoker, total cholesterol 5.0 mmol/litre, BP 130/80†

30 per cent risk of vascular events in 10 years (very high risk)

- 43 years old, male, smoker, total cholesterol 9 mmol/litre, BP 170/90

- 53 years old, male, smoker, total cholesterol 7 mmol/litre, BP 150/90

- 63 years old, male, smoker, total cholesterol 5 mmol/litre, BP 140/80

- 73 years old, male, non-smoker, total cholesterol 5 mmol/litre, BP 140/80

- 53 years old, female, smoker, total cholesterol 7 mmol/litre, BP 180/90

- 63 years old, female, smoker, total cholesterol 7 mmol/litre, BP 150/90

- 73 years old, female, non-smoker, total cholesterol 7 mmol/litre, BP 170/90

---

*If diabetic, this individual would move into the 10–20 per cent risk group.

†If diabetic, these individuals would move into the over 30 per cent risk group.

Calculated using the web-based Vascular Risk Calculator at: http://cvrisk.mvm.ed.ac.uk/calculator/bnf.htm

We will explore these preventative measures by order of risk, so let us first consider primary prevention for low-risk asymptomatic people.

Preventing vascular disease in low-risk asymptomatic people

In Chapter 2, I discussed the important vascular risk factors for stroke (high blood pressure, smoking, diabetes, high cholesterol) together with the other treatable risk factors such as atrial fibrillation. It follows that strategies which lower blood pressure and blood cholesterol, reduce smoking, reduce the prevalence of diabetes, and treat atrial fibrillation will be effective in stroke prevention (provided that such strategies do not have an unexpected adverse side effect). Geoffrey Rose, a renowned British epidemiologist, described the two main strategies very elegantly as a population approach; and a high-risk approach.

Blood pressure provides a very good example of these two complementary approaches. If we consider the blood pressure of a typical population, it follows a bell-shaped curve; in other words, a minority of people have blood pressure readings at the extremes (high or low), and the majority have blood pressure around the average. This is known as a normal distribution curve (Fig. 8.1). Such curves exist for many physiological variables. In medicine we currently arbitrarily define hypertension as a blood pressure above 140/85 mmHg, and the previous focus has been on identifying and treating hypertensives (Fig. 8.1(a)). This is the high-risk approach: screen and identify those at greatest risk of stroke. However, let us see what happens if we shift the entire curve to the left by a small amount (Fig. 8.1(b)). An extraordinary result is achieved: by making a small change in the entire population, we have achieved a large

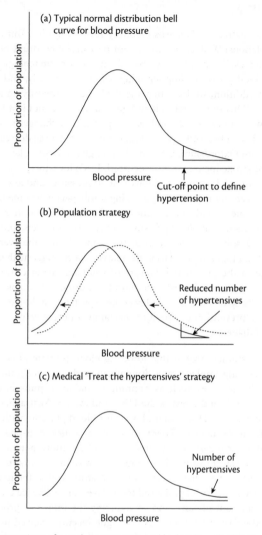

Figure 8.1 Comparison of population strategy and high-risk medical strategy. (a) The blood pressure of a population follows a bell-shaped normal distribution curve. Few people have very low or very high blood pressures. Most have readings about the average. Medically we have defined a level of blood pressure which we consider abnormal and label people hypertensive. (b) If we can move the entire population curve to the left, for example by reducing the population-wide consumption of dietary salt, we can potentially reduce the number of people in the abnormal right-hand tail of the graph (the hypertensives). (c) If effective interventions can be found to cause the effect seen in (b), we can reduce the number of 'hypertensives'.

change at the extremes. This was Geoffrey Rose's big idea. But can we treat entire populations? Well the answer is not necessarily by drugs but by public health strategies. There are ways based on non-pharmacological evidence to reduce blood pressure: stop smoking, exercise regularly, and reduce dietary salt. In addition, we have become far better at identifying and treating hypertension. This sounds all well and good in practice, but is it feasible? The exciting news from recent research is that population changes in vascular risk factors have been observed *together* with the predicted large decrease in stroke. In studies from Oxfordshire, UK, and Framingham, USA, a large decrease in age-adjusted stroke incidence has occurred. In Oxfordshire, it was noted that people presenting with stroke had lower blood pressures and lower blood cholesterol and were more likely to be taking antihypertensive medication than at an earlier time period in the same area. In Framingham, there was also a population reduction in blood pressure and cholesterol levels, and a reduction in smoking. Despite the increase in diabetes and obesity, the overall 'vascular risk' in the Framingham population decreased, which suggests that the favourable change in the potent risk factors of smoking, hypertension, and high cholesterol will overwhelm the bad news from obesity. Perhaps this explains why the obesity epidemic has yet to lower life expectancy in developed countries. However, the prevention of obesity is certainly a potent way of reducing the incidence of diabetes.

If population studies suggest that lowering blood pressure, lowering cholesterol, and reducing smoking rates dramatically reduces stroke, then the recent public health measures such as banning smoking in pubs in Ireland and Scotland (and now in the rest of the UK), and even in Australia, is great news for stroke prevention. How can we lower our blood pressure without recourse to tablets from the doctor? There are many so-called non-pharmacological methods, and salt ingestion is probably one of the more potent hypertensive agents that we can do something about. Salt was an essential preservative of food in the days when there were no refrigerators. Today, the majority of the salt in our diet comes from processed foods (even foods like ice cream can contain a large amount of salt), and so reducing the intake of processed foods will help reduce your salt intake. A colleague recently showed me two different brands of tinned tomatoes, and there was 100 times as much salt content in one brand as in the other! The potential obstacle to reducing dietary salt includes the fact that many people complain that food tastes bland without added salt. Indeed, food manufacturers know this, and they add more and more salt to processed foods to get the maximum taste 'hit'. If they overdo it, food will taste too salty, and so they generally go just below that limit. An additional commercial advantage of salty foods is that they make you thirsty, making you more likely to buy and consume soft drinks (which are often full of sugar!). The good news to counter the 'taste' argument is that when you reduce your salt intake *slowly*, you will adapt and food can still remain tasty.

Other non-pharmacological methods to reduce blood pressure are shown in the box. Blood pressure is such an important treatable cause of stroke that treatment with drugs should be initiated for healthy people, who are otherwise low risk, if their blood pressure is greater than 160/100 mmHg and should be considered for those with blood pressure greater than 140/85 mmHg. The treatment of hypertension has been around for so long that much of this medical practice was developed before the days of 'evidence-based medicine' and cost-effectiveness. Therefore we have developed an 'antihypertensive strategy' which routinely treats some people at quite low risk and therefore is very costly (if we consider cost per stroke prevented). However, blood pressure medication is generally so safe, and blood pressure is such an important cause of stroke and other vascular disease, that this is still accepted as reasonable. This practice becomes less evidence based in the very elderly, as antihypertensive medication commonly causes side effects, and there have been far fewer trials. But on the basis that treatment effects rarely reverse in old age, it is reasonable to consider treatment, even in the oldest old (aged over 85 years).

Non-pharmacological methods of lowering blood pressure

- Reduce added salt in cooking and on the table

- Increase foods high in potassium (e.g. bananas, chocolate, coffee)

- Increase regular exercise

- Stop smoking

- Relaxation techniques ('biofeedback')

- Avoid excessive alcohol

- Have a pet dog (good stress reliever and encourages 'walkies')

Blood cholesterol can be lowered by following a low-fat diet. Encouraging people to have at least five helpings of fresh vegetables and fruit a day will help them avoid the other fatty foods in the diet. It is recommended that adults keep total fat intake to 20–35 per cent of calories, and saturated fats less than

10 per cent of calories, with most fats coming from sources of poly- and mono-unsaturated fats, such as fish, nuts, and vegetable oils. Clinical trials have suggested that dietary changes have only modest effects for individuals, but the Framingham and Oxfordshire data indicate that these modest individual effects can produce surprisingly large benefits for the population.

To put all this in perspective, the reduction in smoking has probably had the greatest public health impact for the individual and population. The reduction in smoking prevalence has been a huge public health success in countries like the UK. In just over 30 years, the proportion of adult smokers has halved, and now is about 25 per cent for men and 23 per cent for women, representing about 10 million people. The aim is to reduce the prevalence still further to 21 per cent by 2010 in the UK, and it is hoped that the legislation to reduce smoking in public will be the final encouragement people need to give up this very addictive habit. There are many proven ways to stop smoking for the 70 per cent of smokers who want to give up.

Proven strategies to decrease cigarette smoking

◆ Nicotine replacement treatment (gum, transdermal patch, nasal spray, inhaler, and tablets/lozenges which dissolve under the tongue)

◆ Intensive support for hospitalized patients (better than simple advice)

◆ Simple advice from health professional

◆ Individual or group therapy

Preventing vascular disease in high-risk asymptomatic people

There are now many vascular risk scores which all aim to predict who is most likely to have a stroke (or other vascular event) in the future. At present, there is a consensus that, in developed countries, lifestyle changes (discussed above) and medication are recommended if your risk of a stroke or heart attack is thought to be more than 20 per cent over the next 10 years. If you are in this category, then typical goals of treatment will be to lower blood pressure, and certainly to make sure that it is less than 145/80 mmHg, and to ensure that cholesterol level is generally as low as possible, and certainly below a total cholesterol level of 4 mmol/litre (or below 2 mmol/litre for LDL-cholesterol). It goes without saying that you should be a non-smoker.

There are some risk factors that will quickly take you over the 20 per cent 10-year risk, and diabetes is an example (see box in previous section). The vascular risks for diabetics are so much greater than those for the non-diabetic population that they will often end up in the high-risk category for primary prevention purposes. Appropriate control of blood glucose, together with reduction of blood pressure and cholesterol, is the most effective way for diabetics to reduce their vascular risk.

Secondary prevention of stroke

The first key consideration must be to treat the cause of the stroke (see Chapter 5). For example, if the stroke was due to a rare cause such as infective endocarditis (infection of the heart valve), the best way to prevent further stroke is prompt diagnosis, identification of the bacterial or fungal organism causing the infection, and high-dose intravenous antibiotics (and possible surgical replacement of the damaged heart valve). Similarly, strokes due to vasculitis need treatment for vasculitis. Strokes secondary to illicit drugs needs abstinence from the offending substance (e.g. cocaine). However, these causes are the minority, especially in older people.

For the vast majority of people with stroke of any type (infarct or haemorrhage), two major preventative measures should be universally considered: stopping smoking and reducing blood pressure. These two measures are effective for both ischaemic and haemorrhagic stroke, and the evidence suggests that lowering blood pressure can reduce the chance of stroke by about a third, and probably more for people with primary intracerebral haemorrhage. I am using the phrase 'blood pressure reduction' on purpose because I do not merely mean treatment of hypertension (blood pressures greater than 140/85 mmHg) but also the reduction of blood pressure for those with conventionally normal levels. By the 1990s, it was well established that high blood pressure was a cause of stroke, but it also became apparent that even in individuals with 'normal pressure', a higher blood pressure was associated with a higher risk of stroke. It was then shown that this relationship was also true for survivors of stroke and those with TIA. This set the stage for a large-scale randomized trial which demonstrated that the use of two widely available blood pressure tablets could reduce the risk of stroke by about a third over the next few years. This trial was effectively a 'population intervention' for a population of people who had survived a stroke and thus had a similar effect to that seen in Fig. 8.1(b). It is almost certain that this is not due to any one particular blood pressure lowering agent, but merely requires safe medication with an ability to lower blood pressure effectively. There are a few provisos to this general recommendation. We are not yet sure of the best time to start lowering blood pressure; the

113

trials started treatment in people some weeks and months after their stroke. Secondly, lowering blood pressure lowering can have major side effects in some people, especially older frailer people, as it is a common cause of falls and syncope (fainting). Thirdly, this intervention usually requires medication which adds to the multiple recommended tablets for the stroke survivor.

Additional secondary prevention measures for ischaemic stroke

Antithrombotic treatment

Blood-thinning medication (antithrombotic treatment) should be considered for all patients with ischaemic stroke, i.e. stroke due to thrombosis. The evidence for this is substantial and we can make quite clear recommendations. First, if ischaemic stroke was associated with the common heart rhythm disturbance atrial fibrillation (AF), anticoagulation with warfarin (or a similar coumarin drug) will reduce the subsequent risk of stroke by a massive 60 per cent (see box).

Warfarin

In the 1920s a mysterious illness was causing fatal bleeds in cattle on the prairies of North Dakota and Alberta. This was traced to fermenting hay, from which a new substance, called dicumarol, was isolated. Warfarin was named by Karl Link and stands for 'Wisconsin Alumni Research Foundation ARIN', where 'arin' indicates coumarin which is the generic name of the substance found to be the mysterious cause of the fatal cattle bleeds.

Source: Link KP (1959) *Circulation*, **19**, 97–107

The downside to this major treatment benefit is the problem of anticoagulation. Warfarin has numerous interactions with other drugs, and regular blood tests are needed to determine the correct dose. The dose of warfarin depends on many factors, dietary vitamin K (warfarin acts by acting as a vitamin K antagonist, and vitamin K is required for the production of clotting factors in the blood), age, gender, weight, and genetic factors such as the genotypes of certain genes (e.g. cytochrome P450 2C9 (*CYP2C9*) and vitamin K epoxide reductase (*VKORC1*)). Prediction models have been developed to try and help estimate the required doses (see www.warfarindosing.org) but regular blood tests are still necessary. The important side effect of warfarin is an increase in fatal or disabling bleeds, particularly those causing intracerebral bleeds. In clinical trials, the benefits of warfarin overwhelmed these devastating side effects and there was substantial net benefit. However, we do not know for certain whether warfarin should be continued in extreme old age (although the recent trial results are reassuring), and there are well-known contraindications to long-term anticoagulation (see box).

Typical reasons to avoid using warfarin

Active bleeding

Bleeding tendency (e.g. haemophilia)

Unreliable at taking tablets

Alcoholic liver disease

Falls risk

Extreme old age

Previous haemorrhagic stroke

Despite the problems of warfarin it is quite remarkable that, to date we have been unable to identify a reliable modern equivalent drug despite many attempts to design a better thrombin inhibitor.

Antithrombotic treatment in the absence of atrial fibrillation

Blood-thinning medication with antiplatelet medication should be considered for all patients with ischaemic stroke who are not eligible for warfarin. Again, we have substantial data from numerous clinical trials to guide therapy and a number of different tablet regimens are effective. Historically, aspirin was the first agent to be widely used for this indication. Aspirin reduces the risk of stroke by about a fifth; therefore if your risk of stroke over 1 year is 5 per cent, regular aspirin would reduce this to 4 per cent. Initially the dose of aspirin was similar to the anti-inflammatory or pain-killing dose (1200 mg), but subsequent research has shown that lower doses of aspirin are still effective as blood thinners, with the advantage that the lower the dose of aspirin, the lower the stomach irritation side effects. Whilst a daily dose range of 30–1200 mg of aspirin a day is effective, the best doses are in the region of 75–100 mg a day. The advantages and disadvantages of aspirin are shown in the box.

Advantages and disadvantages of aspirin

Advantages	Disadvantages
Effective antiplatelet agent	Risk of severe allergic reaction in some people (e.g. Asthmatics)
Very cheap	Can cause stomach ulcers and gastritis
Widely available	Increases the risk of haemorrhagic stroke
May prevent cancer (e.g. colon cancer)	Can cause constipation
	Can cause indigestion and heartburn
Cost-effective medication	Exacerbates bleeding disorders
	Can cause skin bruising

Two further blood-thinning medications are effective and widely used. Clopidogrel is also an antiplatelet agent, and in large trials it has been shown to be as good as, if not slightly better than, aspirin when compared head to head. One distinct advantage of clopidogrel is that it does not have the stomach/indigestion side effects of aspirin; however, it causes more skin rashes and diarrhoea. It is widely used as an alternative to aspirin, especially for people who suffer from indigestion/heartburn or stomach ulcers. Dipyridamole is another antiplatelet agent which has been used for decades. It also has a similar benefit to aspirin but, more importantly, two large clinical trials have demonstrated that it can be safely used in combination with aspirin to confer even greater benefits. In general it is a very safe drug, but it can cause troublesome headaches when first started. However, these generally resolve in a few days. Other side effects include some gastrointestinal problems and faints due to postural hypotension. Current evidence suggests that a combination of aspirin and dipyridamole is the best antiplatelet blood-thinning combination for people after stroke.

Combinations of aspirin and clopidogrel have been tested and are not recommended for people after stroke as the bleeding side effects cancel out the additional benefits of preventing stroke due to blood clots. What makes life more complicated in this area is that this same combination (aspirin and clopidogrel) is a standard treatment after heart attacks and coronary stenting. The reason for this discrepancy between stroke medicine and cardiology is that the risks of a vascular event in the 6–9 months after a heart attack are somewhat greater than those after stroke, and thus the aspirin clopidogrel combination has a net benefit in the cardiological situation despite very similar risks for combination treatment. This example illustrates the complex balancing of risks and benefits of some medications so that the same tablet may be harmful if used in some situations, yet beneficial in others. It certainly does not allow for simple messages – something that is a cause of great frustration for the pharmaceutical industry.

The pharmaceutical industry is very interested in this area of medicine as the potential markets are huge (millions of people treated for many years), and thus there are numerous new trials underway or planned testing better antiplatelet agents or novel combinations of agents. One of the larger trials currently nearing completion is a study comparing clopidogrel with the combination aspirin–dipyridamole; therefore further information in this area will be available soon.

Cholesterol lowering

It is only in the last few years that cholesterol lowering has become widely used to prevent strokes and other vascular events following an ischaemic stroke. There are several reasons for this: effective cholesterol lowering agents (the 'statins') have only been developed in the last few decades, the epidemiology of cholesterol and stroke was not clear (see Chapter 3), and large trials of cholesterol lowering drugs specifically looking at stroke patients and including older people, have only recently been completed. However, we now have clear evidence that the lower the blood cholesterol (within a surprisingly large range), the lower is the subsequent risk of ischaemic stroke and other thrombotic vascular diseases (such as heart attack), and the statin group of medications are very safe and effective. In fact statins are so safe that simvastatin is available without a doctor's prescription in the UK. Because of the cost of these drugs, cholesterol lowering has been quite an expensive way of reducing stroke risk, but as the older statins come out of patent, cholesterol lowering is becoming increasingly cost effective. In general, it is best to use the highest tolerated dose, as a lower blood cholesterol is associated with a lower vascular risk. One interesting quirk of the cholesterol story is that many of the previous randomized controlled trials had an age limit of 75 years (an age limit that would exclude about half of all people with stroke). This was done because of a misinterpretation of the epidemiology of cholesterol and disease in older people.

One influential study found that the relationship of cholesterol to heart disease deaths was significantly positive at ages 40, 50, and 60 years but attenuated with age until the relationship was positive, but not significant, at age 70 years and negative, but not significant, at age 80 years. Although the authors of this study advised that this question would need to be addressed by appropriate randomized controlled trials, the medical community acted by imposing an age limit of 75 years in many of the cholesterol lowering trials that followed. The influential Heart Protection Study was one of the first to include older people, and evidence from this and subsequent trials has demonstrated that older people stand to benefit as much as, if not more than, younger people from cholesterol lowering. Therefore cholesterol lowering should be considered for all patients with ischaemic stroke, no matter their age, to help prevent future vascular disease. In contrast with this historical ageism, another problem to emerge from modern secondary preventative treatment is that doctors are sometimes reluctant to stop treatment when many would argue that it is no longer worthwhile. As a geriatrician I see many severely disabled frail older people admitted to hospital from nursing homes on numerous medications, including statins, and their admission has often been precipitated by drug side effects. The message should be that all secondary prevention should be reviewed from time to time, and it may be very reasonable to stop some treatments depending on the clinical situation and the wishes of the patient and family.

In general, cholesterol lowering drugs should not be used for people who have had a haemorrhagic stroke as there is currently no evidence of benefit and a potential risk of further haemorrhagic strokes.

To summarize the preventative measures discussed so far:

- all stroke survivors should try and improve their lifestyle (good diet, avoid smoking, regular exercise)

- blood pressure lowering and avoiding blood-thinning medication such as aspirin is important for those who have had a stroke due to a bleed

- blood pressure and cholesterol lowering, together with some form of blood-thinning medication (anticoagulation for those in atrial fibrillation, antiplatelet therapy for the rest), is recommended.

We will now discuss some of the more complicated stroke preventative strategies.

Carotid intervention

Carotid stenosis causes stroke due to the formation of platelet emboli on the atheromatous lining of the artery (e.g. when the atheroma has split or fissured), and breaking off. The arterial blood flow carries the emboli to the brain, blocking a cerebral artery and causing an ischaemic stroke. The other mechanism of stroke from a carotid stenosis occurs when the stenosis occludes, thus blocking all flow through that carotid (one of only four major blood vessels to the brain). Treatment of carotid stenoses can prevent future strokes. Intervention includes the following:

◆ surgically removing the atheromatous plaque (**carotid endarterectomy**)

◆ opening the stenosis with a catheter (**carotid angioplasty**)

◆ opening the stenosis and covering the abnormal plaque with a stent (**carotid stenting**).

Carotid interventions are effective stroke preventative measures for both asymptomatic people and those who have already had a stroke or TIA, but this is a complex area and patient selection is crucial as the procedures carry a significant risk.

Carotid interventions for asymptomatic people

> Carotid endarterectomy with any less skill than exhibited by ACST and ACAS surgeons quickly casts the procedure into the list of 'risk factors for stroke.
>
> Henry Barnett, *Lancet*, **363**, 1486–7, 2004

This quote from Henry Barnett nicely encapsulates the problem with carotid endarterectomy for asymptomatic carotid stenosis. Two large trials (ACST and ACAS) have demonstrated that surgery can be effective, *but* there are some important provisos. First, the risk of stroke for people who did not have surgery in these trials was only 2 per cent per year, and there is reason to consider that this low risk could be reduced further by more intensive vascular preventative measures (antiplatelet therapy, cholesterol, and blood pressure lowering treatment, avoiding smoking, and adopting a healthy diet and exercise programme, as described above). It is unlikely that all these strategies were used to their maximum effect for the participants in these trials, especially as some of the new data showing the benefits of cholesterol lowering were only emerging as these trials were nearing completion. Secondly, the risk of surgery was remarkably low in these trials (a 3 per cent risk of peri-operative stroke or death), and audits have demonstrated that it is difficult to achieve these low risks in routine medical practice. Thirdly, in public health terms, many people have to undergo surgery to prevent one stroke, making it a very expensive medical treatment. However, many countries (and individuals) are now rich enough for this not to be a major problem. Finally, there is the problem of risk: some people are more comfortable taking an early risk of surgery to reduce their subsequent risk of stroke, while others would rather avoid surgery and take their chance. This is a complex area and patients are likely to do best in a large carotid surgery centre with a multidisciplinary team of stroke physicians, neuroradiologists, and surgeons.

Carotid intervention for symptomatic individuals

Symptomatic people are those who have had an ischaemic stroke or TIA in the territory of the abnormal carotid. This immediately declares three issues: there needs to be an accurate diagnosis of stroke or TIA (not always easy), brain imaging needs to have excluded a bleed as a cause of the symptoms, and clinical assessment and/or brain imaging information is required to determine whether the event is likely to be a carotid territory event. Even when these three issues have been resolved, the question of treatment is again complex! The balance of risk and benefit differs as follows.

- Degree of carotid stenosis: a tighter stenosis confers a greater risk of subsequent stroke.

- Gender: women have less to gain from surgery.

- Delay from initial event: the benefit of surgery declines with increasing delay from the initial stroke or TIA.

- Potential risks from investigations: catheter angiograms used to be performed routinely to assess the degree of stenosis, but this test can cause stroke!

- Increasing surgical risks can negate the benefits of the procedure.

- Surgical techniques can influence effectiveness: issues include the use of a patch to repair the artery, whether the surgery is performed under local or general anaesthesia, and whether a bypass procedure is employed.

- Non-surgical techniques are available but are not definitely superior to a surgical endarterectomy; carotid stenting is technically feasible and may be preferred by some patients and doctors.

Despite this daunting list of issues, carotid surgery offers an excellent method of reducing the high risk of subsequent stroke for carefully selected patients. It is certainly not a cheap preventative measure, but in the right hands it is very effective. The key aspect of success is to ensure management by a good multidisciplinary group of stroke physicians, neuroradiologists, and vascular surgeons.

Summary

We now have the knowledge to prevent most strokes, but as countries and individuals we still do not have the will. The great success at reducing stroke incidence in parts of the UK and USA has only just managed to keep total stroke incidence static because our populations continue to age into the really high stroke risk period. In other parts of the world, increases in cigarette smoking and other vascular risk factors, together with an ageing population, will predictably lead to more and more people having strokes. My hope for the future is that stroke services and research will start to receive a larger share of health resources to lead a new war on stroke with effective implementation of prevention together with better treatment, rehabilitation, and care for stroke survivors.

Further reading

Antithrombotic Trialists' Collaboration (2002) Collaborative meta-analysis of randomized trials of antiplatelet therapy for prevention of death, myocardial infarction, and stroke in high risk patients. *British Medical Journal*, **324**, 71–86.

Collins R, Armitage J, Parish S, Sleight P, and Peto R; Heart Protection Study Collaborative Group (2004) Effects of cholesterol-lowering with simvastatin on stroke and other major vascular events in 20 536 people with cerebrovascular disease or other high-risk conditions. *Lancet*, **363**, 757–67.

Cook NR, Cutler JA, Obarzanek E, *et al.* (2007) Long term effects of dietary sodium reduction on cardiovascular disease outcomes: observational follow-up of the trials of hypertension prevention (TOHP). *British Medical Journal* **334**, 885.

ESPRIT Study Group, Halkes PH, van Gijn J, Kappelle LJ, Koudstaal PJ, and Algra A (2006) Aspirin plus dipyridamole versus aspirin alone after cerebral ischaemia of arterial origin (ESPRIT). A randomised controlled trial. *Lancet* **367**, 1665–1673.

He FL and MacGregor GA (2002). Effect of modest salt reduction on blood pressure: a meta-analysis of randomized trials. Implications for public health. *Journal of Human Hypertension*, **16**, 761–70.

Link KP (1959) The discovery of dicumarol and its sequels. *Circulation*, **19**, 97–107.

PROGRESS Collaborative Group (2001) Randomised trial of a perindopril-based blood-pressure lowering regimen among 6105 individuals with previous stroke or transient ischaemic attack. *Lancet*, **358**, 1033–41.

Rose G (1992) *The Strategy of Preventative Medicine*. Oxford University Press.

Rothwell PM, Eliasziw M, Gutnikov SA, *et al.* (2003) Pooled analysis of individual patient data from randomised controlled trials of endarterectomy for symptomatic carotid stenosis. *Lancet*, **361**, 107–16.

Glossary

Activities of daily living (ADLs) basic activities required to exist in a reasonable state

Aneurysm balloon-like swelling in the wall of an artery

Aphasia problem of language production and understanding

Apoplexy ancient name for devastating stroke

Atheroma narrowing of blood vessels due to build-up of abnormal arterial wall material

Atrial fibrillation (AF) irregular and uncoordinated beating of the heart

Brain attack new name to describe the typical features of stroke and transient ischaemic attack in the first 24 hours

Brain haemorrhage leakage from or bursting of the cerebral artery

Brain plasticity brain reorganization to allow previously dormant or under-used regions to take over functions damaged by the stroke

Brainstem the base of the brain containing all the nerve fibres from the spinal cord

Carotid endarterectomy removal of atheroma

Carotid stenosis narrowing of the carotid artery in the neck

Carotid syphon disease narrowing of the carotid artery within the skull

Catheter flexible tube for introducing or removing fluids through a narrow opening

Cerebral artery blood vessel in the brain

Cerebral infarction death of brain tissue

Cerebral thrombosis clots in the blood vessels in the brain

Cerebrovascular accident alternative term for stroke

Circle of Willis circle on the undersurface of the brain formed by linked branches of the arteries supplying the brain

Cochrane Library electronic archive of systematic reviews of randomized controlled trials of thousands of different interventions

Cognition mental functions carried out by the human brain

Cryptogenic stroke stroke without an identifiable cause

Dissection internal splitting of a blood vessel wall

Dysaesthesia unpleasant sensation sometimes felt when an area of the body weakened by stroke is touched

Dysphagia difficulty swallowing food or water

Embolus a blood clot which has travelled along the blood vessel from a source further away

Epidemiology branch of medicine that deals with the incidence, distribution, and control of disease in a population

Haematoma volume of blood in a primary intracerebral haemorrhage

Haemorrhagic transformation of infarction bleeding associated with a cerebral infarct

Hemianopia loss of visual field on one side

Hemiparesis (hemiplegia) paralysis of the face, arm, and leg on one side of the body

HMG-Co A reductase enzyme which increases the production of cholesterol in the body

Hypertension high blood pressure

Iatrogenic disease illness due to medical intervention

Incidence of stroke how many new strokes occur each year

Intracranial haemorrhage abnormal blood within the skull

Ischaemic stroke stroke caused by blood supply to the brain (occlusion)

Lacunar infarction (LACI) strokes due to blockage of end-arteries; they eventually leave a small hole (lacuna) in the brain

Lumen space within a blood vessel

Metabolic syndrome high blood cholesterol, high blood pressure, and diabetes

Myocardial infarction heart attack

Nasogastric tube feeding tube placed in the stomach through the nose

Neurons brain cells, also known as grey matter

Occlusion blockage of blood vessels, usually by a blood clot

Oedema excessive accumulation of fluid

Oxfordshire Community Stroke Project (OCSP) classification system for classifying ischaemic stroke

Partial anterior circulation infarcts (PACI) milder version of a TACI in which the arterial occlusion is further downstream and thus affects a smaller volume of brain

Percutaneous endoscopically placed gastroenterostomy (PEG) tube feeding tube placed through the stomach wall

Posterior circulation infarct (POCI) large stroke due to occlusion of the posterior circulation

Prevalence of stroke how many people are alive having survived a stroke

Primary intracerebral haemorrhage (PICH) stroke caused by brain haemorrhage

Primary prevention of stroke efforts to prevent stroke in people who have not had a stroke

Prothrombotic states conditions that thicken the blood

Risk factors for stroke characteristics (of an individual or population) that are associated with an increased risk of stroke compared with those without those characteristics

Secondary prevention of stroke aims to prevent a second, or subsequent, stroke

Spasticity increase in tone during muscle movement which can lead to spasms, flexion contractures, and limitations of movement

Sphygmomanometer instrument for measuring blood pressure

Statins drugs which inhibit HMG-Co A reductase and reduce blood LDL-cholesterol

Subdural haematoma bleeding around the brain

Thrombolysis breaking up blood clots

Thrombophilia genetic predisposition to 'thick blood'

Total anterior circulation infarct (TACI) large stroke due to occlusion of a large blood vessel of the brain

Transient ischaemic attack an ischaemic stroke with symptoms lasting for less than 24 hours. Also known as a 'mini-stroke'

Unilateral hemiparesis weakness down one side

Vascular disease disease of the blood vessels

Venous sinus thrombosis blood clots in the veins that drain the blood from the brain

Appendix

Stroke helplines and resources in the UK, Australia, and the USA

USA

Stroke Association

http://www.strokeassociation.org/

Call 1-888-4-STROKE (or 1-888-478-7653)

Australia

The National Stroke Foundation: http://www.strokefoundation.com.au/; Tel: 1800 787 653.

UK

The Stroke Association: http://www.stroke.org.uk/; Tel. 0845 3033100.

Chest, Heart Stroke Scotland: http://www.chss.org.uk/; Tel. 0845 077 6000

Different Strokes (a charity set up by younger stroke survivors for younger stroke survivors): http://www.differentstrokes.co.uk/

Afasic: http://www.afasic.org.uk/

Speakability: http://www.speakability.org.uk/

Other useful websites

Stroke Prevention Research Unit, University of Oxford: http://www.stroke.ox.ac.uk/

Vascular Risk Calculator: http://www.cvrisk.mvm.ed.ac.uk/calculator/bnf.htm

World Health Organization: http://www.who.int/whosis/mort/profiles/en/index.html

World Health Organization: http://www.who.int/en/

Index